DISCLAIMER AND TERMS OF USE AGREEMENT:

(Please Read This Before Using This Book)

Read all my books on Kindle for free without downloading or printing except you want to buy them.

Contents

How To Manage Irritable Bowel Syndrome (IBS)

Overview Of Treatments For IBS

Is Stress A Factor For IBS?

Dieting And Its Effects On IBS

Understanding The Medications For Treating IBS

Treatments For Irritable Bowel

Preventing Irritable Bowel By Managing Stress

What You Can Do To Improve Your Irritable Bowel

Living With Irritable Bowel

Alternative Treatments For Irritable Bowel

Cats Irritable Bowel

Causes Of Irritable Bowel Syndrome

Signs Of Irritable Bowel Syndrome In Children

Common Diets For Irritable Bowel Syndrome

Diarrhea, The Symptoms Of Irritable Bowel

Diet For Irritable Bowel: What-To-Eat And What-Not-To-Eat

Diet Suggestions For Irritable Bowel Syndrome

Tips On Preventing Feline Irritable Bowel Syndrome

Irritable Bowel Syndrome + Neuroendocrine

Facts About Irritable Bowel Syndrome

Irritable Bowel Syndrome

Alternative Healing For Irritable Bowels

Irritable Bowel Diet

Important Facts On Irritable Bowel Diet

Irritable Bowel Disease

Irritable Bowel: Why It So Often Goes Untreated

Are You At Risk For Irritable Bowel?

Understanding Irritable Bowel

Are You Suffering From Irritable Bowel?

Why Irritable Bowel Can Hurt You

Irritable Bowel Triggers

Seeking Medical Attention For Irritable Bowel

Irritable Bowel: Understanding What Happens At The Doctor

Diagnosing Irritable Bowel

Irritable Bowel: What's The Worst?

Effects Of Smoking On Irritable Bowel Syndrome

Healing Irritable Bowel Syndrome The Natural Way

The Seven Sins Of Irritable Bowel Syndrome Diet

Irritable Bowel Syndrome Online

Constipation And Irritable Bowel Syndrome

Irritable Bowel Syndrome – General Information, Treatments And Causes

The Use Of Zelnorm To Treat Irritable Bowel Syndrome

What You Should Know About Irritable Bowel Syndrome

Diagnosis And Treatments For Irritable Bowel Syndrome

What Is Irritable Bowel Syndrome?

Common Irritable Bowel Syndrome Symptoms

Understanding Irritable Bowel Syndrome

Treatments For Irritable Bowel Syndrome

What Is Irritable Bowel Syndrome

How To Manage Irritable Bowel Syndrome (IBS)

Irritable bowel syndrome is something that no one really wants to talk about, but more people need to hear about.

This condition affects an average of 50% of those that visit the gastroenterologist each year. Even if you haven't gone there yet, it is likely that at some point, you will want to make the journey.

The condition is one that is likely to cause you a great deal of pain and discomfort. For that reason, it is imperative to learn all that you can about what irritable bowel syndrome is as well as how it can be relieved. That's what we aim to do here. But, before you can find relief from irritable bowel syndrome, you must know what it actually is.

What Is It?

IBS, as it is called for short, is also known as spastic colon. In this condition, individuals will experience pain in their abdomen. The pain is due to a disorder of the function of your bowel. In addition to pain, you may also experience changes in normal bowel habits.

IBS Symptoms

The most frequent symptoms include:

- Pain in the lower abdomen
- Bloating
- Pain that is relieved by defecation

If you are suffering from any of these conditions, you may want to talk to your doctor, especially if they are recurring.

Overview Of Treatments For IBS

Irritable bowel syndrome is not something that has a 100 percent cure rate. In most cases, you and your doctor will work at determining how best to tackle and handle the symptoms. Without the cause being known, there is little that can be done to remove the pain and discomfort forever once and for all.

One thing that should be noted is that irritable bowel syndrome is not a progressive condition. It is also not life threatening to those that suffer from it. There is no reason to believe that you can't get help and will have to suffer with IBS either.

But, there is much that can be done to help in improving the quality of your life by handling the symptoms that you face. That is what we'll provide here.

How To Manage IBS

There is a lot to think about when it comes to managing IBS. There are medications, home remedy solutions and other things that you will need to do to help you to stop the pain and suffering that you are experiencing.

In most cases, you can get some relief by implementing just one of the types of treatments available to you. But, most that suffer from IBS will want to consider doing more than just adding one treatment to their regimen for managing IBS. With a constant eye on several key factors, you can find a number of benefits in health related costs.

Treatments To Be Considered

There are several types of treatments that can be used in the relief of irritable bowel syndrome. In later chapters, we will go into full details about each of these so that you can adapt them into your lifestyle and find the relief that you need.
- Stress relief

- Your diet
- Prevention of the condition

Is Stress A Factor For IBS?

Stress is most definitely related to causing your IBS to get worse. It will irritate IBS and make things more harmful!

One of the first things that you and your doctor will talk about in regards to your IBS is that of stress. Stress if a factor that can do damage to many aspects of your health including irritable bowel syndrome.

First and foremost, don't make the mistake of thinking that stress in and of itself can cause IBS. This is not the case. Stress is generally brought into our lives by a troubled lifestyle. The more stresses that you put onto your body, the less healthy and capable of producing a healthy reaction it is.

Remember that we don't know what actually causes IBS. In effect, all we can do is to treat the symptoms that can come from it. But, we do know what makes it worse and stress is one of those factors.

Why Stress Hurts

The facts on why stress hurts your IBS are clear. For a healthy person in an ideal situation, stress is controlled by the body. Your body has a pain inhibition system that turns on when it is struggling with pain to help you to cope with it.

But, what has been found in patients with IBS is that this hypersensitivity doesn't go away. Your body doesn't turn on the right pain inhibition system and you feel the muscles of your gut hurting.

For example, it has been a long and stressful day, you are looking forward to a good meal and sleep. If you are experiencing prolonged or repeated episodes of stress, you'll find it not so easy to relax. Instead, you go home and eat a meal. No matter if you eat during your stressful event or after, your will have that awful ache in your abdomen that comes with IBS.

This would be a normal feeling of being full for some, but for those with IBS it hurts. Your body doesn't turn off the pain function that a healthy body would which in turn allows you to feel more of the pain associated with eating during or after stress.

Dieting And Its Effects On IBS

We talked about stress being a big factor for IBS. Now we will talk about another big factor for agitating IBS and that's your diet.

Like stress, your diet does not bring on IBS. Although many people thing that they have caused this condition by eating less than healthy foods, that is not the case. Yet, it is well known that foods can contribute to making irritable bowel syndrome worse.

The problem with food is double. First, your body may react to some foods in a more intense way with IBS than others would react to that food. In addition, the body experiences increased levels of intestinal muscle reaction and sensitivity with IBS than otherwise. Just the fact that you are eating can make the symptoms of IBS show themselves. It may not even be a specific food that is causing it, but a general overreaction to food.

The Problems With Foods

The first thing to work on is the simple fact that you can control what you eat. In that, you can have some control over how your body reacts with IBS symptoms. Some of the foods that we know are problematic for those with IBS include foods like fried foods, alcohol, caffeine and foods that are high in fat. In addition to this, when too much food is consumed at one sitting, problems can also arise.

Diarrhea and cramping in your abdomen can be caused by some specific types of sugars that are unable to be fully digested by the bowel. These include sorbitol which is a sweetener in dietetic foods, gum sugars, candy sugars, and fructose. The consumption of these sugars will lead to the inability of the bowel to absorb them correctly and will lead to diarrhea.

The gas symptoms of IBS can be brought on by some foods as well. For example, beans, legumes, cauliflower, lentils, Brussels sprouts, onions, bagels, cabbage and broccoli all can

How To Win Your War Against Irritable Bowel Syndrome

bring on more intense gas like symptoms of IBS. Eating these types of foods can bring on the symptoms of IBS including bloating and increased gas.

With these foods being behind the onset of symptoms of IBS, it is important for you to consider how they affect you. It is essential for you to understand that foods affect each person in a different way. What affects you and causes intense symptoms of IBS is not the same and doesn't have the same effect on another person with IBS symptoms. For that reason, it is critical that you find out how foods affect you.

Understanding The Medications For Treating IBS

Irritable bowel syndrome is a condition that has several medicinal choices for relief. In most cases, these medications are not given to everyone, but to those with a moderate to extreme level of IBS symptom severity. In other words, they may not be the right choice for you.

These medications come in several forms and you may have heard a lot about them when you visited your doctor to become diagnosed with IBS in the first place.

If your doctor did not mention them, or you are not sure if they are right for you, talk with your doctor. Your individual situation may warrant a different medication or just lifestyle changes to meet your symptoms.

It can't be said enough that the most benefit to managing IBS symptoms comes not from medication treatments, but rather from the use of lifestyle and dietary changes in your every day life. Making changes to your stress levels helps as well.

If these changes are not enough, then you may be eligible for medication. For those individuals, let's break down the options that are available to them.

The First Line

The first line of medications is over the counter. In many cases, your IBS symptoms may be mild and for them there is no need for prescription treatment. Some of the medications and treatments that may be helpful to you include these:

·   ***Fiber supplements.*** As we mentioned earlier, fiber is a critical part of maintaining health. In the case of IBS, the right amount of fiber is required to provide the individuals with necessary help in relieving constipation. Fiber supplements may be the best route to this. There are two types. Psyllium which is like the brand name Metamucil and methylcellulose which is like the brand name of Citrucel.

· **_Anti Diarrhea Medications._** These are medications for the opposite effect. They will work to control diarrhea. You can purchase loperamide such as the brand name Imodium to help with the diarrhea that your IBS symptoms may produce.

<u>Treatments For Irritable Bowel</u>

There are many ways that your doctor will help you to improve your health through the management of your irritable bowel syndrome. Doctors don't know what the cause is of it and they don't have a specific medication that can make it go away. There is no cure for IBS. But, there are many things that you can do, including a handful of treatments that can, ultimately, improve your quality of life and limit the symptoms that you face.

Those that have mild symptoms of irritable bowel syndrome will work closely with their doctors to determine any triggers that cause it to come on. They will make changes in their lifestyle as well as managing their stress better that will improve their chances of avoiding serious problems with IBS. Yet, those that have more severe problems may need some additional help. Your doctor may provide you with that help in a number of ways.

- Fiber supplements may help to control your constipation and may be recommended to help make you regular.
- Medications for diarrhea control are also likely to be used to help control diarrhea to keep you hydrated.
- You may make dietary changes that will help to lessen the amount of gas that your body produces.
- Medications such as anticholinergic and antidepressants may be used to further treat your condition. Anticholinergics are medications that help to relieve the spasms that happen in the bowel that are very painful. Antidepressants are used to help those that suffer from depression as well as pain.

Each person is likely to experience a different type of condition as they go through irritable bowel syndrome. For that reason, you and your doctor will work closely to determine the best course of action for your specific case. Then, your treatment plan can be effective.

Preventing Irritable Bowel By Managing Stress

If you are experiencing the pains of irritable bowel syndrome, you probably need to seek the help of a doctor to help you to find ways to manage your condition. But, there is likely to be help for you through prevention as well. Those that are struggling to find improvements in their health can often do so by just learning a few ways to manage stress, one of the leading reasons that people struggle with irritable bowel syndrome in the first place.

There are a number of ways that you can improve your condition by learning to manage the stress that you are under. Here are a few helpful tips for making sure that happens.

1. **Seek help for your problems.** If you have constant levels of stress, counseling or having an outlet can help to relieve that stress enough that your body can improve physically. You need to learn how to reduce your stress and counseling can be one of the best ways to make that happen.
2. **Practice relaxation experiences.** Things like yoga, massage and meditation also help to relieve stress. If you find that you need some way to relieve it, try one of these low key ways of making it happen. You may be surprised how easy stress can melt away.
3. **Deep breathing techniques can be taught to you as well.** Learning how to control your breathing to improve your heart rate can help to reduce stress and ultimately help you to feel better. If you learn better techniques of breathing, such as learning how to breathe from your diaphragm, you can prevent many of the problems you face.

Preventing irritable bowel syndrome is something that you should do. It's something that can help you to avoid the countless problems that you face each day due to this condition.

<u>What You Can Do To Improve Your Irritable Bowel</u>

There are actually many things that you can do to improve your irritable bowel syndrome right from home and right now. Although you should work with a doctor to determine what your condition is as well as anything that can be found that is causing it, ultimately much of the management of this condition will need to come from you. The good news is that it can be easily to improve your IBS with a few of the various techniques listed here. Even more so many of those that suffer from this condition find long term relief from IBS by using any of these methods.

Make these changes in your lifestyle to improve your overall health and ability to deal with irritable bowel syndrome.

- ***Learn to avoid problems especially when it comes to the food you eat.*** With your doctors help you'll be able to learn what foods and other consumed products you take in effect your irritable bowel syndrome. By working together, you can determine what could possibly be wrong as well as ways to improve your overall health. But, most importantly, you'll learn that some foods are just foods you need to stay away from. Doing so stops them from bothering you.
- ***Eat normal sized meals regularly.*** Learning to eat at the same time every day can help you to improve your digestion and ultimately will reduce the IBS symptoms you have. This will help to regulate your bowel function, making it easier for you to predict what's going to happen.
- ***Learn to manage your stress.*** This is one key element in improving your IBS. By reducing stress, you reduce the amount of episodes that you face.

When you learn to make changes in your lifestyle like these, you can learn to have more control over your irritable bowel syndrome. The fact is that managing IBS is something that you can tackle.

<u>Living With Irritable Bowel</u>

In the worst case scenario, irritable bowel syndrome can be one of the most devastating conditions because it limits the things that you can and can not do. If you are suffering from this condition, they you already realize that there are ways that you can manage it. If you don't know this, you should learn as much as you can about IBS so that you can improve your overall health. Living with irritable bowel syndrome doesn't have to be a curse, though. You can learn to manage your condition and improve your quality of life.

One thing to do is to learn as much as you can about irritable bowel syndrome. And, then keep learning. Since there is quite a bit about irritable bowel syndrome that is still left to be determined, it makes sense that ultimately you'll be able to find some answers down the road as researchers begin to learn new things about the causes and the cures of IBS. Keep learning.

In addition, you should keep in good contact with a qualified doctor. Sometimes finding a doctor that specializes in these conditions will be the best route to go, especially if you are one that suffers from it over a long period of time or has severe symptoms. You can keep yourself on pass to find benefits to treatments as well as learning new ways to keep yourself feeling good.

Living with IBS can be something that you have to work on improving. It takes some time. It definitely takes learning a new lifestyle that will improve your well being. Finally, it may take some time to balance out the right treatment that will benefit you more so than others. Living with irritable bowel syndrome is something that you can do. Working towards success is something you'll strive for.

Alternative Treatments For Irritable Bowel

Sometimes, the best medicine for a condition like irritable bowel syndrome is not medicine at all. Today, more people are turning towards alternative treatment options for their health conditions because they are seeking less costly and ultimately fewer side effects. When you consider the many benefits of alternative treatments for irritable bowel syndrome, you'll find plenty of routes to consider. While you shouldn't stop doing what your doctor tells you to do, these treatments are going to play a role in helping you to improve as a compliment to your current treatment.

Here are some treatment options that you should consider.

- *Acupuncture Is one treatment option to consider.* Irritable bowel syndrome can be treated by acupuncture by a skilled technician. You'll find that results vary but that many swear by this treatment. Acupuncture is an ancient Chinese treatment based on inserting needles in specific locations around the body to relieve pressure points. It's been used to treat thousands of people of many conditions.
- *Herbal supplements can be helpful as well.* For example, the herb peppermint may be helpful in relieving stomach pain and discomfort. In addition, it can help to relieve other symptoms like heartburn. Make sure that any herbs you consume do not interact with the medications your doctor prescribes for you, though. Talk to a herbologist for more options.
- *Probiotics are another treatment.* These are good bacteria that live in your body, especially in your intestines that are needed for digestion. By supplementing those that you have, it is believed that they can provide you with some relief. Some people believe that if you suffer from IBS you don't have enough of these in your system.

Those suffering from irritable bowel syndrome have countless benefits available to them through treatment. With the help of your doctor, you can manage IBS with any of these alternative or other treatments. The good news is that you can learn to control it so much so that you don't have to think about it all the time.

Cats Irritable Bowel

If you were under the impression that Irritable Bowel Syndrome occurred only among humans, you are far from the facts since it is common for animals and in particular cats to suffer from it. They experience similar symptoms as humans.

IBS among these four legged felines is also a gastrointestinal disorder as in human beings. Also either the small or the large intestine or both are affected. Irregular movement of bowels is the chief effect of IBS in cats due to contraction of the digestive tracts. Apart from this, the distribution of food and waste in the cat's digestive system is affected. This leads to accumulation of mucus and toxins in the intestines of the cat.

These toxins that accumulate hurdle the proper functioning of the digestive tract. This leads to trapping of gases and stool which in turn causes distention and constipation. It might come in as a surprise to know that human IBS factors have almost the same effect on cats. Stress, poor eating habits, overdose of antibiotics, viral and bacterial infection, food allergies and parasites were found to cause IBS in felines too.

Also since cats like chewing and also swallowing objects, the chance of blockage is high. This is yet another trigger of IBS.

IBS Symptoms in cats:

There are many common symptoms of IBS between cats and human beings. Some of them are presented in the following list.

- Constipation that is often a symptom of IBS. In cats, it is characterized by small, hard, pebble-like stools. This makes movement of bowels difficult.
- Often, diarrhea is common among cats with IBS where the stools are soft and watery. These cats experience alternate periods of diarrhea and constipation.
- Cats also experience mild to severe abdominal pain.
- Mucus mixed with stool is a common symptom of IBS in cats.
- Cats with IBS may also have nausea and may vomit. This is a sure sign of IBS
- Flatulence or pain due to accumulation of gas is an indication you're your cat has IBS.

- Bloating
- The cat cannot tolerate certain food types
- Anorexia is also surprisingly common among our feline friends.

Finding a cure for your cat's IBS

Irritable Bowel Syndrome might be caused by various factors. It is important to zero down on the right one. A vet alone can help you in doing this. He can immediately tell you what triggered IBS in your pet. Even if you prefer using natural methods to control IBS in your cat, consult a vet first so that further complications are avoided. Then continue with your methods with the consent of the vet.

You can control IBS in your cat by changing its diet. Consult a vet or a nutritionist when you decide to make a change so that they can prepare a custom diet program for your pet.

Find the right type of food that agrees with your cat's digestive system. Cats are very similar to humans in the fact that they prefer variety in food. Some like raw food while some others prefer canned food. Certain cats may like home-made food too.

Keep experimenting with your cat's diet till you find one that suits it best. Keep a journal to keep track of the various food items your cat has to avoid. This will help you a lot in the later stages to feed your cat with non-IBS triggering foods and thereby keep IBS in control.

Causes Of Irritable Bowel Syndrome

It is not uncommon for people aged over 20 to suffer from the condition commonly referred to as the irritable bowel syndrome. Though it is very commonly diagnosed people prefer not to discuss this issue with others.

Frequent stomach cramps, abdominal pain, bloating, diarrhea and constipation characterize Irritable Bowel Syndrome known as IBS in short. It leads to a great amount of discomfort and leaves the sufferer in distress though no permanent harm is done.

Though IBS is common among many patients and so are their problems, the symptoms of IBS are varied. This makes diagnosis a bit difficult.

Some of the people suffering from IBS, experience only a single symptom like constipation. This is characterized by straining or cramping with only minimal amount of stool released. Some people experience mucus, which moistens digestive tracts, released in their stool along with bowel.

Some others have more serious symptoms like diarrhea which causes release of watery stools which is both uncontrollable and frequent. Some others suffer from alternate attacks of diarrhea and constipation.

It is wrong to imagine that the syndrome has stopped when the symptoms cease. Some people in fact find irritable bowel syndrome more difficult to tolerate months after the symptoms cease.

Though IBS is reported all around the world regularly, the exact causes of this syndrome have not been determined. Many researchers have come to a common conclusion that it is related to colon and that large bowel may be reactive to stress and food consumed.

Many others believe that inefficiency of the immune system is the chief cause of IBS.

How To Win Your War Against Irritable Bowel Syndrome

These IBS patients also commonly suffer from irregular movement or motility in the large colon. This is referred to medically as spasmodic movement. Some others experience intestinal movement temporarily ceasing.

Bacteria in the gastro-intestinal tracts have also been often linked to the causes of IBS. Researches have observed that people who have previously developed gastroenteritis have an increased chance of developing IBS too.

Irritable bowel syndrome is found to heighten when a person is susceptible to stress and anxiety. This in turn aggravates IBS. Also many IBS symptoms cause anxiety and depression.

Study of some other patients has led to the general opinion that celiac disease and IBS may be interrelated. Celiac disease is a person's inability to digest a substance present in rye, barley, wheat flour and other substances that help coagulating bread called gluten. The immune system of celiac disease patients is affected and it damages the small intestine when gluten is consumed. The presence or absence of celiac disease can be confirmed using blood tests.

However, among female sufferers of IBS, the symptoms were found to get worse in their menstrual period.

These commonly observed factors are the "supposed causes" of movement of bowel internally. There is constant research in the medical and scientific circles for a definite and feasible cure for easing out of this syndrome.

People have found various things that can give temporary relief from IBS. These are mainly centered at avoiding certain trigger foods that can cause symptoms that lead to Irritable Bowel Syndrome. Also there are many activities that are suggested which are known to lessen the effects and chances of appearance of these symptoms. Abstinence from alcoholic drinks, avoiding large means, reducing consumption of caffeine, tea, chocolates and colas and using wheat based food items are recommended.

Signs Of Irritable Bowel Syndrome In Children

IBS of the Irritable Bowel Syndrome is an ailment which mainly upsets the large intestine and the colon. They large intestine, is the component of the human digestive system which accumulates stools. Though the main triggering factor of this is still unknown it has a number of symptoms attached to it which helps in identifying the disorder.

This ailment is comparatively widespread in Americans. The deficiency of proper research regarding this syndrome is one of the major reasons for an effective treatment in not being established. Only very critical conditions are paid attention to while carrying on research activities and as Irritable Bowel Syndrome is just chronic, efforts are not being taken to carry on research in this field. Adding to the misery is the verity that the IBS is a functional ailment which adds to the complication of the need for a treatment which is viable.

Functional disorders are frequently allied with symptoms and sensations which may vary from person to person and thus, cannot be quantified in any terms. For instance, pain cannot be measured and studied under any common scale. In case the Irritable Bowel Syndrome comes along with ulcer, then the damage in the intestinal tissues can be considered as a basis to determine the extent of the ailment.

As the IBS is only a functional disorder, physical symptoms are not common as the syndrome depends more on the functions performed by the human digestive system and more precisely, the colon. The Irritable Bowel Syndrome, both in adults as well as children makes the nerves and muscles of the colon extremely sensitive and any stuff which is beyond the tolerance of the colon muscles would result in the system being extremely affected.

The next factor which makes the situation worse is the lack of absolute knowledge regarding the reason of the Irritable Bowel Syndrome. It may either be constipation dominated Irritable Bowel Syndrome or diarrhea controlled Irritable Bowel Syndrome. The study and treatment for both the types is different.

This state is more common among people who are 20 years of age and above. However, it is likely to be prevalent among children too. In such a case, the symptoms are minimal and milder than that in adults. Very often, aggravated constipation or diarrhea is wrongly concluded as

How To Win Your War Against Irritable Bowel Syndrome

Irritable Bowel Syndrome. Hence, it is important to get a child who is suspected to have Irritable Bowel Syndrome diagnosed by a doctor.

The most noticeable symptoms among children as regards to the Irritable Bowel Syndrome are diarrhea and constipation or a combination of both. There may also be cramps felt in the abdominal area. Diarrhea is the unexpected change in bowel movement frequency. It is characterized by impulsive urge to discharge stool which usually results in incontinence. Easy discharge of fluid-like stool is also considered to be diarrhea. Sometimes, the child may even feel that the discharge of stool has not been complete and would have the impulse for another bowel movement right after.

Parents need to be advised and assisted in the entire process to save their child from any complication. Dehydration may be caused if proper care of the child is not taken. For this purpose, it is highly necessary to consult a doctor.

Alternatively, constipation is the condition in which the stool solidifies so much that it cannot be excreted through the anus. The best alternative in this case is intake of lots of fiber rich food which add weight to the stool.

The important sign in children, of Irritable Bowel Syndrome which can be easily identified is if they have not had proper bowel movements in recent times. Irritable Bowel Syndrome in children is a more complicated situation because if it gets aggravated, it would result in increased discomfort to the child. Hence, its preferable to get it treated at an earlier stage.

Common Diets For Irritable Bowel Syndrome

Keeping track of very morsel of food consumed is deemed to be important by a large number of people with Irritable Bowel Syndrome. Not only do they need to know what they eat, but also the way in which the food was prepared.

For example, if you consume chicken, it is insufficient to just indicate "chicken" in your journal. Instead you need to add the specifics like the time at which you ate and even your mood while eating. By noting down such fine details, you can find out what affects you and what doesn't.

Keep regularly filling your food journal to keep a continuous track of what you consume. The best way to do this is to sit during the night and fill it in so that you don't miss out on anything. Give every detail equal attention and jot it down. Even a very insignificant item like a bar of chocolate can play a huge role in choosing the best diet plan for you.

Eliminating trigger foods is the common root of all Irritable Bowel Syndrome special diets. A dietician or physician can help you lay out a good plan for your weekly/monthly diet. But he must have your food journal to decide this.

In order to eliminate constipation, a common recommend of most IBS specific diets is the addition of a large amount of dietary fiber. Fiber acts as a neutralizer for your food.

When fiber content in your food is high, your stools become bulkier. This increases the volume of your stools. The best way to cure constipation is to counter the compacted stool. Fiber does just this and so is an integral part of most Irritable Bowel Syndrome diets.

Trigger foods or problematic foods are those food items that can trigger or aggravate symptoms leading to IBS. They have high fat content. Fat often takes longer than fiber to dissolve and get assimilated by the human body.

Take meals at regular intervals if you are following an IBS diet. This is because IBS mainly is caused by abnormalities in the intestinal tract and/or the colon. When you eat at the same time every day, your body and thereby your intestine and colon will get used to the schedule and

How To Win Your War Against Irritable Bowel Syndrome

would help regularize bowel movement. Once bowel movement is regularized and intestinal muscles are strengthened, this Irritable Bowel Syndrome ceases.

Consume small meals only if you have Irritable Bowel Syndrome with symptoms of diarrhea. It is recommended that you consult a dietician or a general physician to know how much water you must consume since a lot of water is released in the stool when you have diarrhea.

Consume a lot of fluids if you suffer from IBS. Alcohol is best at this. Be cautious and avoid carbonated soda, caffeinated beverages, and alcoholic drinks. These can further stimulate the intestines and worsen this condition. Carbonated drinks produce gas which also aggravates IBS.

It is advised that people with IBS should avoid all dairy foods. This clause is a part of almost all IBS diets. Use yogurt instead of milk proteins. Use enzymes that can help you break down lactose. This is because most IBS affected people are lactose intolerant.

You can continue consuming milk products. It is however recommended by most IBS diets to eliminate lactose from food. In order to supplement this lactose free diet, consume food that is rich in vitamin B, protein and calcium, so that your body does not miss any essential nutrients.

Diarrhea, The Symptoms Of Irritable Bowel

There are a variety of signs which typify the Irritable Bowel Movement. It might diverge from a mild form to severe symptoms. However, the positive aspect of the Irritable Bowel Movement is, though it may range from mild to acute symptoms, it would never proceed to more severe intestinal problems such as cancer or colitis. The reason behind this is, the non-existence of soreness in the muscles of the intestine and many other conditions which may aggravate the symptoms.

Diarrhea is one of the most common and frequently appearing symptoms of the Irritable Bowel Movement. In some cases, diarrhea may be coupled with constipation. Constipation is set apart by watery or loose stool or the stool may be too condensed to be discharged through the anus.

Diarrhea can be explained as the state of augmented occurrence in bowel movement. It is also characterized by incontinence of stool. Incontinence is nothing but the incapability to restrain or hold-up bowel movement. Also, sudden intense impulse for bowel movement, if not addressed at once may result in incontinence. Partial evacuation may also be felt wherein the individual suffers the need to rush for another bowel movement following the first one. However, the upcoming ones would be tougher to expel.

The most common signs of diarrhea are as described below

Irregularity of stools- this cannot be termed as the characterization of diarrhea. The diet of the person helps in judging the extent to which the individual has been affected. But, this alone cannot be solely relied upon. There are many other factors influencing it too. People who consume lots of fibers, fruits and vegetables have looser stool while the rest have more solid stuff. However, too watery stools are considered diarrheal.

Occurrence of bowel movement- there is no specific rule related to the number of bowel movements which is considered normal. Depending on the routine of the individual, three times a day or three in a week is considered normal. Below this limit is taken as irregular bowel movement. Nonetheless, more than half of the population all around the world observes the one-time-per-day custom as "standard clean-up".

How To Win Your War Against Irritable Bowel Syndrome

However, among people in the pink of health, the appropriate number of bowel movements is five times per day. Anything beyond this is considered diarrheal. Hence, once this level is crossed, they are said to be having diarrhea.

Diarrhea may also be built up due to non-standard level of water content in stool. For the proper digestion process, food is maintained in a liquefied form with the help of the discharge of water from the pancreas, stomach gall bladder and upper small intestines. The remaining undigested food reaches the large and small intestines in liquid state.

After this, the lower part of the small intestine sucks up the water left in the remaining undigested food. It would then turn the undigested food to a more solid form. The absence of this process is another characteristic feature of diarrhea. It may be caused due to excessive secretion of water through the distal end of the small intestine which may result inefficient absorption. In some cases, it may be caused due to quick exit of the undigested food through the intestines resulting in the stool to stay watery.

Diarrhea generally plays a part in the advancement and worsening of the Irritable Bowel Movement. Adequate knowledge about the signs and the nature of the problem would help in prevention as well as cure of the syndrome.

Diet For Irritable Bowel: What-To-Eat And What-Not-To-Eat

The very fact that food plays a role in causing irritable bowel syndrome will not come in as a surprise to many. Everyone knows that it is our intestinal tracts that process food. So the proper functioning of the intestines is dependent on the food we eat.

The fashion in which our body digests food is affected by a drastic change in diet. The chemical interactions that help processing the nutrients in the food are changed by this change in diet.

These interactions alone, or rather the change of them, do not cause irritable bowel syndrome. This syndrome is a functional disorder that is dependent on various abnormalities that may or may not project complications physically. This is why the cause of this syndrome is partly unknown till date. Most of the factors that cause this are subjective in nature and require treatment which is also subjective. This is more than enough proof why there is no concrete knowledge of what causes this.

Though we know what the various factors that contribute to IBS and even find the consequences of this syndrome are, the medical researchers are unable to provide a comprehensive plan for IBS patients.

Any activity directed to removing these factors will lessen the chances of this attack but may not cure it completely.

Follow a diet plan that does not contain these problematic foods. Instead, include food items that can help you make your digestive system healthier.

There are certain foods that don't contribute directly to IBS but have substantial effects. A perfect strategy for creating an IBS-patient-friendly diet is unknown. Normally foods that strengthen the intestinal tract and foods that have lesser chances of triggering IBS must be combined together for the optimal diet.

Foods that cause some tension in the stomach or cause it to malfunction are called trigger foods. These mostly have very low fiber but extremely high amounts of fat. Coconut milk, oil, cream, fried food, poultry food etc are well known triggers.

How To Win Your War Against Irritable Bowel Syndrome

The rate of digestion in the stomach is reduced by fats. The longer it takes for the bacteria in your intestine to consume them. This results in the risk of creating more gas. It is because of this that many people suffer irritable bowel syndrome due to intestinal gases. These gases are also related to diarrhea, constipation, bloating, and other larger complications.

Irritable bowel syndrome is also triggered by highly caffeinated foods like coffee, carbonated drinks, chocolate etc. So if you are suffering from this syndrome or other abdominal complications, eliminate these from your menu.

It is good to consume extra dietary fiber to facilitate smooth movement of stool in the colon. This applies specially to those with irritable bowel syndrome resulting from constipation.

Compact stool or stool that is too loose indicates constipation. Fiber neutralizes this and prevents constipation by adding bulk to the stool and helps the body to expel it.

One can also acquire the necessary amount of fiber from natural resources like fruits and vegetables, figs, brown rice, peas, raisins, French bread, soybeans etc.

Diet Suggestions For Irritable Bowel Syndrome

Irritable bowel syndrome can be characterized by various symptoms having different roots. Therefore it is necessary to find out about each of these roots so that you can be treated better.

It is also quite important that you still are knowledgeable enough of the actual nature if this problem, even if you know the roots of it.

Foods do not cause the attacks of these symptoms. Bloating, constipation and diarrhea are some of the symptoms that can be set off due to certain problematic foods.

Diet patterns differ from person to person. A certain diet plan might work for a person but not necessarily work for everyone. There exists no standard diet for all people suffering from this condition.

However, there are a few foods that have been found to aggravate such conditions.

There is no proper explanation to why certain foods have these effects which trigger on irritable bowel syndrome. The culprit of IBS is what is pointed out to anything associated with the condition towards the specific diet.

The most common placebo among most of the patients is the reduction of these symptoms by the restriction or elimination of those foods that are said to be causing these attacks.

Large meals can cause compaction and strain in the stomach. Hence, it is advised that people should take in many small meals instead of taking three whole huge regular meals. This will surely reduce the triggering of constipation as well as diarrhea.

Fat based foods when reduced by the patients will also help. It is mainly because it is more difficult to break down fatty foods and also it takes longer to digest. Poor digestion is also related to irritable bowel syndrome. Formation of gas in the intestines can further lead to the increase of many more symptoms that can aggravate the problem.

How To Win Your War Against Irritable Bowel Syndrome

The movement of gas is much slower to the small intestine from the stomach when dietary fat is consumed. Quite a number of people seem to have been responding exaggeratedly towards these dietary fats through slowing it down further. As there are not many facts that have been established on this context, it is safer to prevent any of the possibilities from occurring.

The natural components and 'greens' are the best known solutions to most of these intestinal complications. The ill effects of the gastrointestinal tract can be treated by dietary fibers that are got from vegetables and fruits, wheat based products and beans.

Fiber will surely help in problems of constipation even though it might not be helpful in reducing abdominal pain. Fiber increases the bulkiness of stool and hence helps in removing the stool better.

Lactose intolerance is very often associated with this irritable bowel syndrome. Hence people find it very easy to pull away from milk to avoid any other further complications. Lactose elimination will not mean the releasing of IBS symptoms like many other diet plans. It will further add on to the comfort level or lessen the symptoms.

After you know what the things that create these triggering effects are, a diet plan for this syndrome can easily be devised. This will surely not be helpful enough for a treatment. However it will contribute largely to the facilitating large scale plans to suppress these symptoms.

Tips On Preventing Feline Irritable Bowel Syndrome

In cats, the most usual gastrointestinal disorder is the feline irritable bowel syndrome. This happens when the intestinal tract is affected by chronic inflammation.

Only under conditions that are not normal in the contraction of intestines does a cat suffer from this disorder. Mucus and toxins are created in the tool when the normal passage of waste material and food is interfered.

The accumulated material will obstruct the digestive tract of gas and stool. This process results in constipation, diarrhea and bloating.

The causes of feline IBS are unknown. Factors that contribute to it give us ideas on treatment. The exacerbation of these symptoms can be helped by poor eating habits, bacterial and virus infections, stress, viruses and allergies.

The symptoms include diarrhea, abdominal pain, vomiting, constipation, bloating, flatulence, nausea and anorexia.

Cats need to be checked thoroughly by a veterinarian. Cats need to be relieved from these problems though it may not be fatal.

Do feed the cat with the right type of food. It is very important for you to do this. You do not need to follow what other people follow nor do you have to believe in what they think is right or wrong. Needs of the cats differ from ours. Hence they need other forms of supplementation.

Some cats prefer home cooked food while others prefer it raw. Give your cat whatever it feels comfortable with. Most of them are also fine with canned food. Sticking to what you cat feels best is the option you should go for. There exist no specific diets for cats and hence you do not need to stick to a certain pattern of food diet for it.

High concentration of spicy foods, fat in its food, dairy products, sugar and processed foods are substances that can trigger these symptoms. Synthetic preservatives like butylated

How To Win Your War Against Irritable Bowel Syndrome

hydroxytoluene (BHT), ethoxyquin, butylated hydroxyanisol (BHA) and propyl gallate also need to be kept away.

Bottled water can also be used as some cats are sensitive to a few metals in drinking water. Bottled water can be used as a substitute to its fluid.

You need to keep your cat away from parasites. This syndrome is also triggered by parasites which are infested in your cats. Some of the symptoms are vomiting, lethargy, weight loss, loss of appetite, diarrhea, bad breadth, yeast infection skin problems and foul stool odor.

Do not stress your cat. The presence of a few toxins causes stress among cats. Remove all the sources of stress and hence you do not need to bother about it anymore.

For food serving avoid using plastic bowls and cheap ceramic bowls. Attacks from symptoms might also arrive from fumes from bleach, air fresheners, bathroom cleaners and carpet powders. These are quite necessary for those cats which get affected by change in air components.

A few of these measures which are very simple can help in eliminating all the symptoms that might affect your cat. The tips that are stated above may sound trivial but still they create an environment which is much safer and better for your pet.

Irritable Bowel Syndrome + Neuroendocrine

IBS is a disorder due to which patients find changes in bowel habits which may vary from mild to severe conditions. There are no specifically known causes behind IBS because chronic diseases which do not cause risk to life, are not given high priority.

This disorder is largely associated with the malfunctioning of the large intestine, commonly called the colon. Hence, the symptoms are based on this region, and are taken as functional disorders. This simply means that the conditions are not produced by a significant physical problem, but are initiated by the improper functioning of the intestine arising due to stress, strain and negative reactions shown towards food and other substances.

Research studies reveal that IBS symptoms arise after gastroenteritis symptoms subside. Thus, there is possibility of finding internal physical damage on the walls of the intestine, which explains the occurrence of these symptoms in the body.

The neuroendocrine system refers to the working combination of the endocrine system coupled with the nervous system, which are effectively covered and controlled by the central nervous system.

As IBS is directly related to stress factor, researches are being conducted to discover the relation between the working of the digestive system and the functioning of the endocrine system.

The neuro endocrine system possesses complete control over the internal balance state of the body. Hence, it is closely linked with increase in the stress level of the body.

Evidences of high levels of stress on the hypothalamic-pituitary-adrenal region can largely affect the immunity of the body. This explains the sparse inflammation that is often observed among IBS patients. Further, it is observed that stress is the main cause behind aggravated IBS in patients. Hence, it is strongly advised that the patients practice the principles of stress management in order to suppress the symptoms of IBS.

How To Win Your War Against Irritable Bowel Syndrome

As stress is mainly controlled by the secretion of hormones and the internal balance of the body, it is inferred that the neurons and the endocrine system are working towards suppression of IBS symptoms and returning a steady level of balance in the body. Hormones help in manipulation of the level of chemicals, and other specific fluids. They assist in coping up and responding to various situations posed by the surrounding.

Tumors produced by the neuroendocrine cells are called Neuroendocrine tumors. These cells are characterized by the secretion of hormones. The neuroendocrine cells are a part of a network that is collectively called the neuroendocrine system.

Though the neuroendocrine tumors may be identified in several other regions of the body too, it is found that the digestive system has it in maximum number. They are blamed for several symptoms relating to Irritable Bowel Syndrome, including wheezing, flushing of skin and diarrhea. However, all tumors of the neuroendocrine cells cannot be accounted for hormone producers. Only tumors that are labeled as "functioning" are capable of secreting hormones whereas the tumors which are incapable of hormone secretion are called non-functioning or non-hormone secreting tumors.

The neuroendocrine system and hormone secretion are found to have several effects on IBS symptoms and severity levels. But owing to lack of sufficient research on IBS symptoms, many possibilities have not been discovered as yet.

Many medical experts and researchers are praying that once the puzzle is solved, treatment for the symptoms of Irritable Bowel Syndrome can be determined. But at present, we lack sufficient information that can provide suggestions about the final treatments towards the syndrome.

Facts About Irritable Bowel Syndrome

Introduction

Obtained from the word syndrome, it basically means that a collection of disorders causes a major complex condition to arise. It is not known why IBS occurs commonly among middle aged women, and why a specific frequency or intensity of IBS attacks is not experienced among patients.

However, it is considered to be a functional disorder though during examination. no significant sign of colon problem is observed. But, the colon does not work in its usual way. At present, no cause has been identified for the occurrence of IBS, so it cannot be cured currently.

While IBS is a source of mild irritation for some people, for some others, it is an attenuating and disabling feature which affects the normal activities in the person's life.

Symptoms

The Irritable Bowel Syndrome has been found to be closely associated with diarrhea and constipation attacks.

Diarrhea is a state in which one has insuppressible urge towards the release of bowel. It is sometimes matched with the release of mucus mixed with stools.

On the other hand, constipation is a state in which the patient suffers from abdominal cramps, which may or may not be accompanied by release of stool, which is found to be relatively dry and painful.

A number of causes can be held responsible for the development of IBS. It is sometimes found to be associated with intolerable stretching of intestine or disturbance in intestinal muscle movement. If there is no abnormal condition in the anatomy of the intestine, the cause of IBS is said to be triggered by disturbances in the physiology of the body.

How To Win Your War Against Irritable Bowel Syndrome

The commonly observed Symptoms of IBS are listed below

1) Alternative occurrence of constipation and Diarrhea

2) Cramps in abdomen or stomach

3) Bloating of the abdomen

4) Feeling of unfinished bowel

5) Mucus release in stool

6) Gas

It is observed that the intensity and frequency of the above mentioned symptoms vary from patient to patient. So, it is highly recommended that your condition is properly diagnosed by a physician before you take up medications or adopt a treatment plan.

Prevalence

No fixed data is available to give specific information about the number of patients suffering from Irritable Bowel Syndrome. This is mainly because of incidences that are often left unreported and hence do not get documented. However, sources reveal that one out of ten visits to the hospital is related to IBS. It is found the majority of those affected by IBS are women aged above 20 years. However, Irritable Bowel Syndrome may affect any one, irrespective of age.

Though one out of ten visits to the hospital is regarding IBS, most patients are diagnosed only after the condition aggravates. People tend to assume that it would not affect their daily affairs. Further, it is considered to be a psychological issue and not one of physical significance.

The main advantage of IBS is that it cannot develop into a more aggravated condition, owing to absence of factors like inflammation of intestinal walls, bleeding, damage of the colon, and other related cancerous developments.

Though there is some fundamental treatment forth Irritable Bowel Syndrome, it does not guarantee complete cure. As a matter of fact, due to lack of substantial information regarding the disorder, there is no definite cure for the Irritable Bowel Syndrome.

How To Win Your War Against Irritable Bowel Syndrome

Experts highly recommend change in lifestyle, and utmost care regarding intake of food. Another common suggestion is that stress management principles must be implemented as it is directly connected with Irritable Bowel Syndrome.

Irritable Bowel Syndrome

Cause for lack of treatment on Sore Bowel Syndrome

The Irritable Bowel Syndrome is a condition identified by abnormal activities in the large intestine or colon. The exact cause for this abnormal condition cannot be defined as it is only a syndrome. It is also demarcated by symptoms closely connected to the intestinal tract.

Although it is a common condition among the people of America (nearly 15% of the public are affected by mild to severe Bowel Syndrome), sufficient studies have not been conducted to locate the source of this problem. However, it is a functional problem, which justifies why it was initially termed as a disease connected with psychological disorder.

Functional disorder is a state in which no actual complications or grievances are identified during examination. This does not indicate absence of the disorder. Instead, it indicates that the disorder lies in the functioning of the colon.

This implies that the muscles and nerves connected with intestinal activites are not functioning correctly. These nerves do not refer to those located in the digestive system alone, but the brain and the spinal chord are also largely involved.

The various terms that can be used to replace Irritable Bowel Syndrome are spastic colitis, mucous colitis, spastic colon and several others. However, these conditions are found to be very different compared to the disorder described in Irritable Bowel Syndrome.

As the medical community has no in depth reports regarding the causes and symptoms of Irritable Bowel Syndrome, it is highly probable that there are no existing cures for the disorder. At this stage, the best option to treat the disorder is to suppress the pain and aggravation caused during the panic attacks.

The topic of treating Irritable Bowel Syndrome is dreaded, as not many drugs in the market were studied to bring about effective treatment. Further, some of the drugs which have been studied show very low substantial use owing to several reasons.

How To Win Your War Against Irritable Bowel Syndrome

Medical experts lack understanding of the disorder, as it is not life threatening. It is noted that, only disorders which pose a threat to the life of the patient are considered worthy of research studies. In the case of Irritable Bowel Syndrome, the medical community lacks fund for research If financial help is offered, it will effectively contribute towards gaining comprehensive knowledge about the disease.

Additionally, it is found that this disorder deals with subjective states more than objective states. Subjective factors are not reliable as there is no significant data on which researchers can base their study.

The occurrence of subtypes adds on to the complications involved in finding a suitable treatment for Irritable Bowel Syndrome. The subtypes such as Diarrhea-dominant IBS and constipation-dominant IBS are found to gather their sources for different physiological disorders. Hence, chances are high that a drug which is effective for one person may not have any effect on another.

As Irritable Bowel Syndrome is prominently based on subjective pains, it may pose a high risk when it reacts with placebos or inactive drugs. As a matter of fact, research reveals that one third of patients suffering from Irritable Bowel Syndrome produce positive reaction on using drugs which are inactive.

The final inference is that the physiological processes involved in Irritable Bowel Syndrome have not been researched thoroughly. Hence, effective treatment cannot be recommended depending on these mechanisms connected with it.

Alternative Healing For Irritable Bowels

Irritable bowels are quite disturbing to normal life. The fact that it cannot be cured is more of a pain than the fact that it is not at all fatal. These symptoms associated with this bowel problem needs immediate attention and are uncomfortable for sure.

People try to get a cure either by the traditional ways or some of them do try out the modern way to check if it does help by any chance. But, however there do exists alternate ways of healing.

1.   **Acupuncture** – This type of art is based on knowledge of the energy of life. It is known as Qi. It is pronounced as chi. the imbalance or blockage in a person Qi can cause illness to that person. Acupuncture aims at removing this blockage by the use of needles that are small in size. These help in stimulating different pressure points in the body of a person. This helps in balancing the persons Qi.

Acupuncture induces relaxation and relieves stress. People wonder how piercing needles into ones body can help cure pain and also relieve stress. But, however this is said to cause no pain at all. This is because the sizes of the needles are extremely small and are painless. You could go in for acupressure if you are scared of needles. This process uses massaging instead of putting in needles through your skin. It stimulates pressure points and the nerves.

2.   **Herbs** – herbs help in relieving bowel trouble. Many people believe that certain herbs are very beneficial in relieving some of the symptoms of this syndrome. There are two types of herbs which help in treating these symptoms.

a.   *Teas* - Herbs are generally used to make tea. They are steeped or boiled in hot water. The enzymes and the nutrients that can soothe this symptom of irritable bowels are got by steeping. Thus, by drinking tea you are assured to get these nutrients that you will need. Different types of herbs are used to make tea. This improves the flavor as well as the efficacy of the tea.

b.   *Capsules* – many types of herbs are also taken as capsules. These may contain oils of different plants as well as essential nutrients.

How To Win Your War Against Irritable Bowel Syndrome

Why is encapsulation necessary? This is because oil can be irritating to the digestive system. It triggers symptoms of bowel disorder before it nears the stomach. Thus by coating it, the nutrients will go directly to the intestine and work there. It hence helps in relieving pain without causing irritation.

3. **Hypnosis** – a person's state of mind can affect the irritable bowels. People undergo hypnosis to get a proper mind set so that they can control their symptoms without much trouble. This helps in releasing stress and also tries to get a control over the sub conscious mind. This treatment works for people with mild irritable bowel syndrome.

Irritable Bowel Diet

Many people today suffer from an illness called Irritable Bowel Syndrome or the IBS. It is no fatal illness but has a huge effect on one's lifestyle. It is mainly because of the fact that the symptoms of this Irritable Bowel Syndrome need quick attention when it affects a person. A proper diet can ensure you some control over this syndrome. Not many like the name "irritable bowel diet" so let's stick to "a diet for irritable bowel syndrome"? It sounds better one feels.

A person tends to observe these things about food when they suffer from this syndrome:

1. A look of few goods might trigger symptoms of this syndrome. By knowing that certain foods can aggravate their bowel system; people tend to stay away from them. This is one method where one can avoid them.

2. A few types of food are ok to eat. Usually the ones suffering from this illness tries to locate and identify foods that do not cause any harm to them. When they find such foods, they try to substitute this for their normal food they had earlier given up.

3. Some of the foods are totally unpredictable. When you think it might not cause much trouble to your bowel system, it can have adverse effects and worsen the condition. Some maybe used to a type of food, but they often realize it late that it might not suit them. At the same time, a few types of food will have no effect on a person. They blame it on luck.

It is mainly because of the latter that people are hesitant to choose and try and right kind of diet. Most of them are asked to try and find their own personalized diet to help control their syndrome.

There are certain rules that people can follow to find the right diet for their syndrome. The tips given below are certain to aid you to find the right choice of diet.

1. Soluble fiber: when you include soluble fibers in your diet, it helps to prevent diarrhea and constipation. It stabilizes the activities in the gut and stables your system. Since soluble fiber is advertised to be one type of laxative, people are hesitant to add them in their diet. However, one must realize that soluble fibers ought to be included in the diet as it provides stability to the body and prevent the syndrome from affecting you.

2. *Try to eliminate these foods from your daily diet.* Even if you are tempted to, it is better you don't take them.

a.   alcohol
b.   high fat
c.   red meat
d.   caffeine
e.   carbonated food
f.   dairy

3. *Enjoy while you eating food rather than just swallowing it for the sake of it.* Though irritable bowel diet can be a hard thing to follow, try to enjoy it. Do different combinations in your diet to suit your mood. Think of all the ways where you can substitute you're given up foods. Try to understand that thinking of all the food you cannot have can only leave you in despondency.

4. *If you seem to be doubtful about any food, do not try eating it.* Don't blame it on luck if you are affected by it later. Keep in mind that the irritable bowel syndrome is no easy thing to handle. Ask yourself questions frequently to abstain from foods which can cause harm to you. "Is the taste of the food going to help my case?"

Important Facts On Irritable Bowel Diet

Irritable Bowel Syndrome or the IBS is a very common disorder which affects the intestines of a human being. Stomach pain, cramping, gas, bloating and certain discrepancies in your bowel habits are the main symptoms of this syndrome. Diarrhea and constipation are the other symptoms that people can go through when they have the syndrome while some tend to go through both. Fiber rich food introduced into the body at a decent pace can help o control this syndrome. It might trigger the IBS symptoms if fed at a fast rate.

Patients suffering from this syndrome are asked to add high fiber and low-fat food in their diets. This can certainly keep the constipation at check. Fiber of around twenty to thirty grams is ought to be included in one's diet to control IBS symptoms.

Fiber-rich foods and a lot of fluids are essential to keep the IBS symptoms at bay. Grains such as bran, fruits, vegetables, cereals and certain whole-grain breads are rich in fibers. Soluble fibers found in peas, oats and beans help to control diarrhea and constipation.

A few words of advice for IBS patients: It is always better to purchase food after reading the food labels to check if the breads or cereals are made from whole-wheat or whole-grain. If you go for non-vegetarian foods, choose oatmeal, kidney beans, black-eyed peas, bran pinto and kidney beans for rich fiber content. The Cereal you purchase has to contain at least five grams of fiber in it.

In case you are handling gas pain, purchase a few anti-gas pills to counter it. Plenty of fluids have to be consumed to control gas pain. Doctors usually recommend eight glasses of water or any liquid in a day's time. You might take in fruit juices and decaf drinks to keep yourself away from gas pain.

Also keep in track of our IBS symptoms when it strikes you. Have a record of all the foods you take during that time and make sure you do not try eating them again. If you can maintain a food diary, you can to some extent control IBS.

Simple things like dividing your food into smaller meals than having them at one go can help your case to fight the IBS. Multi vitamins and mineral supplements, especially the ones

How To Win Your War Against Irritable Bowel Syndrome

recommended by the RDI, have to be taken to control this syndrome. It is very essential to consult a doctor or a dietician before starting any medication to control IBS. Before you start taking fiber supplements ensure it with your doctor that it will not cause any harm to you.

Try to avoid eating more by eating your food at a slow pace. This can help the food to digest well inside your system. Enjoy your food rather than taking them as a routine. Abstain from alcoholic and caffeinated beverages as they can cause diarrhea.

Irritable Bowel Syndrome outbreaks

Low residue or low-fiber diet is suggested during IBS flare-ups. There are foods you have to consume to control diarrhea and loosen up your stools.

IBS patients resort to different types of food to relieve diarrhea. They even try adjusting the food temperature to help their case but they have to keep in mind that it might not work for every IBS patient. A few find that it works out while many think it doesn't. Before you try out any new methods to keep diarrhea at bay, consult a doctor.

Irritable Bowel Disease

You are quiet mistaken if you think are suffering from a disease when you acquire the irritable bowel syndrome. It is a popular misconception when people tend to think that way. By thinking this way, they aren't doing themselves any good as they affect themselves psychologically.

The term "Irritable bowel disease" if coined in a negative sense can have effect on a person. People often use this term without knowing how it can actually affect a person psychologically. It can be very deceiving to people already going through this syndrome more than the ones who have absolutely no knowledge about this syndrome. They can get easily bogged down by calling it a "disease". It is always better to call it a syndrome when you are in their company.

When people hear the term "irritable bowel disease" they think it is something which causes an epidemic. This is enough for them to avoid the ones who struggle with the syndrome. It is understandable, though, that people do not want to acquire this syndrome and want to stay as far as possible from it. The mentality of the common man is to think that he should stay away from people who are suffering from the "disease", which is actually a mere syndrome. This isn't good for the society. They try to evade from the person and not have contact with him. So this boils down to the situation where the people suffering from this syndrome not only have to go through the symptoms of it but also take the pain of social isolation.

Being socially isolated can be the most hurting thing for a person. Everyone likes to be respected in the society. When you turn out in the public and people think badly of you, it can be very hurting.

In fact, the term "irritable bowel disease" can give other ideas as well; that there can be a cure. But as a matter of fact, this syndrome doesn't really have a cure. So far doctors haven't got their foot down to solve this syndrome.

A person suffering from this syndrome can never take a false hope from anyone. It can be very misleading and deceitful. If they fall for any drugs given to them, the symptoms could get worse.

It can affect their mind so much that they forget how to keep away the symptoms. They usually have several methods to keep this syndrome at bay. They take the methods for granted when they come to know that what they have is curable. It is sad to see people falling for this trap and at the end of the day not feeling any different.

By coining this syndrome as a "disease" can even change the life of a person. It is matter of misquoting which can have long-term effects on a person. So try to avoid using any fancy terms. A syndrome is nothing but a condition plus a given set of symptoms. Try not to avoid people suffering fro this syndrome. Lend your support and have a few encouraging words for them. Do not make them feel uncomfortable.

Irritable Bowel: Why It So Often Goes Untreated

If you suffer from irritable bowel syndrome, chances are that you know something is wrong but you haven't gotten any help for it. This happens often to many people that are struggling with irritable bowel syndrome. The fact is that many people just don't like to talk about it. That is a problem, too, because the pain that comes from it is intense and it can lead to many additional health problems if it is left untreated. The good news is that there is help for those that suffer from irritable bowel syndrome and if its you, you can get help for it fast.

Who's Got It?

It is estimated that one in every five American adults suffers from irritable bowel syndrome. That is millions of Americans that often do not get the help that they need for this problem. The fact is that it is one of the most common types of disorders facing individuals that have to do with digestion. If you suffer from this condition, chances are that ten to twenty other people that you know are suffering too. Most of them don't get to the doctor.

Today, doctors see more and more cases of Irritable bowel syndrome than every. But, if you look back just a few decades ago, you may not have seen this at all. IBS, as irritable bowel syndrome is often called, actually was thought to have been a condition that wasn't a physical condition. It was believed that it was a psychological disorder instead of being physical. This leads to even more people not getting the help that they needed. Over time this can be one of the largest mistakes that you can make.

Irritable bowel syndrome is characterized by bloating, gas and constipation. Diarrhea can also play a role in IBS. The chances that happen in your bowel movement are what can cause this condition. The fact is simple. If you suffer from these symptoms you should seek out the help of your doctor to get the relief that you need and that you deserve. For most people, finding relief is fast and easy. What's more, it is likely that your doctor has seen many cases of IBS and your case won't bother him one bit.

Are You At Risk For Irritable Bowel?

There are millions of people, some place along the lines of one person out of every five that face irritable bowel syndrome. These individuals are not just individuals that have an upset stomach or are worried so much that they feel ill. Irritable bowel syndrome is a factor that affects them because of problems with the internal organs, namely the intestine and colon. If you feel that you are suffering from irritable bowel syndrome, you should seek out the help of your doctor to find the relief that you need and that you deserve.

Some people are more likely to develop irritable bowel syndrome than others. In fact, women are the largest risk group. If you suffer from irritable bowel syndrome and you are female you are far from alone. Two times as many women face this condition as men do. In addition, it seems to affect younger people more so than older people. This may be due to lifestyles that are being lead during this time or simply the amount of hormones that are in the systems of younger people.

Some people that have irritable bowel syndrome report that there are other people in their family that are suffering from similar problems. This could show that it could be a hereditary factor but that's not always the case. In addition, there is no link as of yet that could clearly define this. Therefore, if you and your family are suffering from IBS, it could be related or perhaps not. Both should seek the help of a doctor.

Risks You Can Control

Although you can't control the risk of getting or having irritable bowel syndrome, you could potentially be able to control some of the factors that cause episodes to come on. For example, you and your doctor will determine if there are any foods or dietary changes that need to be monitored so that you can avoid having a reaction to them. By doing this it can help to improve the amount of time between spells of irritable bowel syndrome.

Working closely with your doctor and reporting any potential health concerns that you have will help you to make the right decision about irritable bowel syndrome. Although you can't control the risk factors that play a role in weather or not you suffer from this condition, you can, ultimately, improve your health.

<u>Understanding Irritable Bowel</u>

Those that suffer from irritable bowel syndrome are likely to find themselves struggling with problems that start as abdominal pain and discomfort and can include change in your bowel function. If this could be something that you experience, you should seek out the help of your doctor. Did you know that one in ever five Americans suffers from this condition? And, that one out of every ten visits to the doctor account for irritable bowel syndrome? With this knowledge you should feel confident that your condition is not unlike that of many other people. There is some help in that fact too.

IBS Is Unique

Sometimes people don't want to seek help for their irritable bowel syndrome because they are worried that it could be something worse, something that could lead to a life threatening condition. Yet, doctors estimate that most people that suffer from this condition actually only have a very mild case of it. Even more so, those that do suffer from an intense flair up of IBS can still find help that can improve your health overall. Irritable bowel syndrome isn't like many other diseases that affect this area of the body. Unlike ulcers, ulcerative colitis and Crohn's disease, irritable bowel syndrome is not a condition that will lead to cancers like colorectal cancer, which these other conditions often can be a pre-sign of.

There Is Good News

There is good news that you can definitely count on. For most individuals that suffer from irritable bowel syndrome, the condition can be closely monitored as well as managed with just the help of improving your diet. You can increase your symptom free days when you are able to manage your lifestyle and your stress levels. Through the monitoring of these three things, virtually everyone can improve their condition and leave a relatively improved life.

If you are seeking the help of a doctor for your irritable bowel syndrome, don't rely on medications to improve your condition. Instead, realize that the best treatment for your condition is the treatment of managing your lifestyle. Treatments can help improve your life considerably. You don't have to suffer from a condition that is painful and embarrassing. You can seek help and improve the quality of your life.

Are You Suffering From Irritable Bowel?

Irritable bowel syndrome is one of the most common types of medical concerns today. Although many don't like to admit that they go through this illness, they suffer in silence. Learning the signs and the symptoms of irritable bowel syndrome can help you to understand if this is the type of illness that you are facing. Sometimes, seeing what these symptoms can be can help you to understand exactly why you need to visit your doctor.

What Are The Signs?

Millions of American adults suffer from irritable bowel syndrome. Someplace along the line of one in every five adults suffer from IBS. Here are some of the signs and symptoms of the condition that you may be experiencing. You should realize, though, that many of these conditions can change from one person to the next.

- Pain in the abdomen or cramping in this area.
- Gas, sometimes quite intense and painful, flatulence
- The feeling of being bloated, or retaining water
- Diarrhea or constipation. For many, this symptom will go from one extreme to the next.
- Mucus in the stool

Most individuals that have IBS actually only suffer from mild symptoms that come and go. You may experience these symptoms on and off or you may experience a constant cycle of events. In either case, even mild symptoms can be disabling and limiting to those that have irritable bowel syndrome. Some individuals will have symptoms that don't respond well to the treatment that they offer to fix it. You may take an over the counter medication only to find that the medication has not provided you with the help and relief that you need. In addition, irritable bowel syndrome can often be a symptom of another health condition, and one that could be more serious. For this reason, you need to seek the help of your doctor to determine if there is a potentially worse situation happening.

If you have these symptoms now or they come back time and time again, they you could be suffering from irritable bowel syndrome. Its important for you and your doctor to rule out any other condition that could be causing you to feel like this. Once that is done, your doctor can help you to develop a plan of treatment to ultimately improve your condition.

Why Irritable Bowel Can Hurt You

Irritable bowel syndrome is something that you think you are suffering from. If in fact you are, it should be understood that medical treatment needs to be sought in order for you to improve your health and your well being. The problem with irritable bowel syndrome, though, is that no one knows exactly what causes it to happen in individuals. Although this is frustrating news to the many that want to know what's going on with their bodies, the good news is that doctors and researchers are always working on finding ways to improve their knowledge of this condition.

When you suffer from this condition, the walls of your intestines are affected. Your intestines actually are lined with a muscle mass that is used to help move food. They contract and then relax again in an effort to push the food through. But, unlike a normal person, the person that suffers from irritable bowel syndrome often faces muscles that don't contract and relax in a normal rhythm. In addition, they often have contractions that are stronger or those that have a longer time period that they are in place. If you do have this then food can move through the intestine too quickly, which will then cause gas and other symptoms like bloating and diarrhea. Sometimes, though, when food can't get through because of this muscle reaction, then you could find yourself constipated.

What's Behind It All?

Although doctors are not sure what is actually behind these muscle problems, they do have theories. For example, some researchers find that irritable bowel syndrome is caused by the changes in your nerves that ultimately control the sensations in your muscles and therefore control the contraction rhythm of your bowel. Or, it could be that hormones lie behind some individual's conditions since it is more likely that a woman will experience IBS than a man. Even still, it could be that your central nervous symptom may be causing a problem with your colon.

For many that suffer from irritable bowel syndrome, the reality is that seeking help is a must. By getting help from your doctor, you can help to track when IBS happens to you so that you can, ultimately begin to learn to control it. For many individuals, this means lifestyle changes in stress and in their diet.

Irritable Bowel Triggers

Although doctors don't know what is behind the reaction that your body experiences that causes irritable bowel syndrome, many realize the importance of finding success in treating it. One way for them to do this is to monitor the triggers that are often behind the condition. The mechanics behind irritable bowel syndrome are often not understood by doctors. They don't know what is happening within your body that causes these reactions, but they do know that there are certain things that seem to trigger an IBS episode. By understanding what these triggers are, you can often find relief from the condition.

What Triggers Trigger Your IBS

For most people that have irritable bowel syndrome, there are some things that cause a severe reaction, which is what is called a trigger. For many, this means an increase in things like pressure, gas and pain. These reactions happen because of the reaction that your intestine may have to the trigger. Usually, there are a handful of things that can cause this for you. Whenever you consume anything that works as a trigger for you, the end result is that you feel bad.

Here are a few things that can be considered triggers.

- ***Foods are the most common.*** When you eat a specific type of food, you may experience a reaction to that food. For example, this happens to many that drink alcohol or eat foods like milk and chocolate. When they consume these foods, they may face an episode of either diarrhea and/or constipation. Some researchers believe that you may have a unique food allergy to these foods and that is what causes your reaction to them.
- ***Medications.*** Some that need to take medications of specific types can find themselves dealing with an episode of irritable bowel syndrome. If you find that this is happening, the end result is that you will ultimately experience irritable bowel syndrome.
- ***Stress.*** For those that are under a lot of stress, this too can become a trigger for your IBS symptoms. Those that become under a lot of stress end up facing more frequent problems with IBS.

If you have any of these types of reactions, your irritable bowel syndrome can be helped by reducing the times when this affects you. With the help of your doctor, you can learn what your triggers are and end up getting the help that you need.

Seeking Medical Attention For Irritable Bowel

Although there are millions of people that suffer from irritable bowel syndrome, it is estimated that only half of them actually get the help that they need. Unfortunately, many find that the conditions is embarrassing and don't want to face what the doctor will tell them. Yet, even if you are concerned about your condition just a bit, seeking the help of your doctor can be one of the best decisions that you make. Gathering information about the condition only shows you that there is a need to seek treatment for your condition so that you can find help. In addition, your condition is going to be somewhat different from the next patient. Getting the help you need, specifically is important.

Do You Need A Doctor?

There are actually many reasons that you may need to seek the help of a doctor to improve your health and well being. Here are some of the reasons that you should consider doing this.

- Your doctor can help you to determine if you actually are suffering from irritable bowel syndrome or if there is a possibility of another condition that you could be suffering from. Sometimes the symptoms of IBS are also similar to symptoms of other conditions, which could pose a more serious health risk.
- Your doctor will help you to determine the right course of action for treating your condition. By considering how severe your case is, he or she may recommend treatments that could put an end to your condition.
- Your doctor will help you to determine what your triggers are. Most people face triggers which are, ultimately, a risk factor for increased episodes of irritable bowel syndrome. If you are suffering from episodes of IBS that are triggered by something, your doctor can help you to determine what that is. This way, you can improve your diet to stop these triggers from affecting your life.
- Finally, your doctor is able to insure that nothing happens as a complication of your condition. Those that face increased amounts of pain and discomfort could find themselves with additional health problems down the line.

If irritable bowel syndrome is affecting you, seek the help of your doctor so that you can overcome the symptoms and improve the life that you lead.

Irritable Bowel: Understanding What Happens At The Doctor

You are suffering from pain in your abdomen that you think could be irritable bowel syndrome. You aren't sure but you definitely are feeling embarrassed. Even worse, you realize the importance of getting medical attention for your condition. What you may be worried about, though, is the fact that you don't know what will happen when you do get to the doctor. First of all, realize that every one in ten appointments that the average doctor has is a condition dealing with irritable bowel syndrome. Most doctors deal with hundreds of these cases each year. He knows what's causing it and he can help you to deal with irritable bowel syndrome.

What Happens

When you go to see your doctor for irritable bowel syndrome, chances are good that he will ask you a few questions and run a few tests. Most doctors will give you an overall physical exam and will talk to you about the way that you feel. From this information, he can rule out other conditions. From this point, he's likely to run a few tests.

•   Stool studies are likely to be the first thing that you requests. During these studies, your doctor will screen the stood for malabsorption problems as well as infections. By checking your stool, he can determine possibly what is causing your condition.
•   Your doctor will run a test called a colonoscopy. During this test, your doctor will insert a small, flexible tube which can be used to check the colon for any signs of problems.
•   A CT scan may also be used. During this type of procedure, your doctor will use x rays to determine the way that your internal organs are working. By focusing on your abdomen, he or she can determine if there is a potential problem there.
•   A flexible sigmoidoscopy may also be done. This test will be used to examine the lower part or your colon. A lighted tube that is very flexible is used to determine this.

In addition to these tests your doctor is likely to run blood tests as well as a lactose intolerance test. By looking at the results of all of these tests, he or she can determine if you are actually facing irritable bowel syndrome or if there is a potential for another condition to be causing your pain.

Diagnosing Irritable Bowel

Determining if you have irritable bowel syndrome is an important part of the process of getting help. Sometimes it can be difficult to say for sure that your condition is irritable bowel syndrome and not one of many other gastrointestinal problems. Yet, with the help of your doctor and a few tests, your doctor will be able to tell you if he believes that you suffer from this condition. The good news is that there is a way to determine if this is the type of illness that you are suffering from.

Tests First

The first thing that your doctor will do is run a series of tests to give him something to consider. By taking samples of your stool as well as talking to you about your symptoms and running a few other tests on you, he will have a clear idea of what is happening within your body. Although it may take some time to come to this conclusion, it will happen. The problem that doctors often face with irritable bowel syndrome is that they have to go through a process of elimination to determine if what you have is what he thinks it is. By ruling out other problems, he can come down to IBS and then make a decision.

What Helps Him Make A Diagnosis?

There are actually several key things that must be met in order for a doctor to tell you that you have irritable bowel syndrome. First, he will need to determine that you have been facing these symptoms for at least 12 weeks. Those weeks do not have to be consecutive, though. If you have been having pain in your abdomen and having experience diarrhea, then this meets one of the criteria for being irritable bowel syndrome. Yet, there are other things that must also be met.

Doctors also require that you have two of the following conditions as well as the 12 weeks. You may have a consistency in your stool, for example moving from solid to being soft or the frequency of that stool production. If you have the need to empty your bowels but you can't do so or you have an urgency to do so, this could be another reason. Mucus in your stool is yet another and the final one is bloating or distension in your abdomen. When two of these four things fit as well as the 12 weeks, your doctor is likely to determine that you are suffering from irritable bowel syndrome.

Irritable Bowel: What's The Worst?

Irritable bowel syndrome or IBS is a condition in which you feel cramping and pain in your stomach and experience a number of different problems with your bowel. Those that face a problem with irritable bowel syndrome often do not seek the help that they need to treat their condition. Most often, this is done because of the fear of being embarrassed of talking to the doctor or admitting that you could have a potential problem. When this is the case, you do need to see the doctor because ultimately it will help you to determine what can be done to improve your condition.

When you don't see the doctor, though, there are things that may happen to you do to your irritable bowel syndrome. For starters, you could risk dehydration, which is a common problem for those that experience bouts of diarrhea. In addition to this, you could face eating problems and disorders that stem from your problems eating foods that are safe for you.

Probably one of the largest problems that you will face if you do not seek help for irritable bowel syndrome is that of emotional stress. Many of those that face this condition have stress and emotional problems over it. You simply don't understand what could be wrong. You don't feel like you can go out in public with the way that you feel. You may also not feel that you can handle what's happening to you in terms of pain and discomfort. Mood swings and sometimes even depression can surface because of irritable bowel syndrome and its effects on you.

Most that suffer from irritable bowel syndrome limit themselves because they are afraid of something happening and not having a location to relieve themselves. They often pull out of social activities for fear of embarrassment or having to explain themselves. For these reasons, many don't live life the way that they could potentially do so.

The good news is that with the help of your doctor, you can learn ways to manage your condition and ultimately improve it. You'll also learn how irritable bowel syndrome can be something you don't need to think about often. Seeking help from your doctor is one of the best things that you can do if you suffer from irritable bowel syndrome

Effects Of Smoking On Irritable Bowel Syndrome

Irritable bowel syndrome (IBS) is a disorder that affects the colon, which is also known as the large intestine. The person may experience abdominal pain, cramps, bloating, gas, diarrhea or constipation. Irritable bowel syndrome is also known as spastic colon, mucus colitis or functional bowel disease. It is not a life-threatening disease, nor is it cancerous or contagious. The disease causes discomfort and stress, disrupting daily activities and often affects the sexual life of the patients.

Smoking worsens the symptoms of Irritable bowel syndrome. The symptoms of IBS are worsened by tobacco and it does not matter whether the tobacco is chewed, smoked or inhaled. The fact is that tobacco is a very potent gastrointestinal tract irritant, a carcinogen and a stimulant. Patients suffering from irritable bowel syndrome have a sensitive gastrointestinal tract and are therefore very susceptible to some stimuli that may include certain foods, tobacco, caffeine and alcohol. Of all these stimulants, tobacco is probably the worst.

In general, smoking and tobacco affects all the parts of the human digestive system. It is the biggest cause for cancer. Smoking causes heartburn and reflux, the two triggers for symptoms of irritable bowel syndrome. Smoking also damages the esophageal sphincter causing the acidic contents in the stomach to flow upwards into the esophagus.

Ulcers are caused by the helicobacter pylori bacteria; however, peptic ulcers are caused due to smoking of tobacco. Smoking prevents healing of the ulcers causing it to recur more often. The reason for this is that smoking aggravates the ulcer perforation tenfold. Besides triggering irritable bowel syndrome and causing ulcers, smoking increases the possibility of Crohn's disease and lead to the formation of gallstones.

Nicotine found in tobacco has addictive properties and is a toxin that tends to weaken the esophageal sphincter. This leads to the increased production of acid in the stomach and reduces the generation of sodium bicarbonate that is important in counterbalancing the stomach acid.

Besides nicotine, tobacco contains about four hundred toxins and forty three carcinogens.

How To Win Your War Against Irritable Bowel Syndrome

These harmful substances are carried by the bloodstream to the digestive tract, thus triggering IBS symptoms. Inhaling tobacco smoke can cause gas, belching and bloating that are symptoms of IBS.

Smoking is known to cause cancer of the colon, the kidney, bladder, stomach or pancreas. Long term smoking increases the likelihood of colorectal cancer. The carcinogens in the tobacco smoke enter the colon and tend to increase the polyp size which may lead to cancerous growth. Studies have shown that twelve percent of colorectal cancers are due to smoking.

As we all know, smoking is injurious to health. Smoking increases the incidence of irritable bowel syndrome and can lead to more serious diseases like cancer. Thus, for the sake of your health, quit smoking and lead a healthy life.

Healing Irritable Bowel Syndrome The Natural Way

Irritable bowel syndrome or IBS is a disorder of the colon and is triggered by factors like consuming the wrong type of foods, stress, smoking, alcohol etc. IBS is not a disease but a disorder wherein the bowels do not function properly. It is not a severe disease like cancer or brain tumor. However, it causes severe discomfort and may disrupt the daily life of those suffering from it. About 15 to 20% of the American population suffers from this common disorder. IBS is also known as mucous colitis, spastic colon, nervous stomach or irritable colon. Medication, therapy and counseling are the usual methods to cure the symptoms of IBS. However, medication is not the only way to control the symptoms of irritable bowel syndrome; it can be healed using natural methods too.

Irritable bowel syndrome is classified as a functional disorder, affecting the physiological function of the body. Hence, it cannot be diagnosed in the usual manner by x-rays or blood tests. The symptoms are not clear and the patient may experience either diarrhea or constipation, both contradictory to each other. The causative factors are also not defined and it may affect people with a sensitive gastrointestinal tract. Treatment may involve medication, a change in diet and use of natural means. Some of the natural methods of healing for irritable bowel syndrome are given below.

Colonic Massage:

Colonic massage can be performed while sitting on the toilet or by lying down and bending the knees. Using the fist of the right hand, gently massage the colon by making a circular, digging motion with the knuckles. Start with the lower right side area of the abdomen and work upwards under the right side of the ribcage. Repeat the same process with the left side and also massage the pubic bone or groin area. The main aim of this exercise is to bring on a bowel movement. This exercise relieves colic in newborns, though minimal pressure must be used in their case.

Mind and body healing:

The symptoms of IBS may cause mental and emotional stress to those suffering from this disorder. In order to control irritable bowel syndrome, it is important for the patients to find a

How To Win Your War Against Irritable Bowel Syndrome

release for the mental stress and seek out therapy that uses emotional release. Somato (or body) emotional release is based on the belief that trauma or pain is stored in the body tissues apart from the mind and soul of the patients. In order to heal effectively, these pains should be eliminated from the body. There are various therapies dealing with somato-emotional release and these include craniosacral reiki and acupuncture apart from other energy healing exercises.

Fiber rich food:

Health experts generally advise on the benefits of consuming fiber rich food to maintain a healthy body. However, persons suffering from IBS reap greater benefits by including fiber in their diet. This should be done slowly to avoid any further complications. By observing what kind of foods agree or don't agree with your digestive system, you can avoid the incidence of irritable bowel syndrome. It is advisable to keep away from foods that trigger an attack of IBS.

The Seven Sins Of Irritable Bowel Syndrome Diet

Irritable Bowel Syndrome or IBS is a disorder of the gastrointestinal tract and related to the colon. Food habits play an important role in the incidence of irritable bowel syndrome apart from other factors. The diet specified by the doctors for those persons suffering from irritable bowel syndrome is crucial because consumption of some foods may trigger the attack of IBS in them. One needs to stick to the diet and the eating guidelines given by doctors because this may be the only way to prevent future symptoms. However, there are some general guidelines related to food that may help to keep irritable bowel syndrome at bay. There are seven such guidelines that may be strictly followed by those affected by IBS:

1.   *Coffee:* Coffee has become a very popular drink and most Americans depend on it to give them the energy to go through the stressful day. They are habituated to drinking endless cups of coffee and damaging their health in the process. Coffee is a known trigger for an irritable bowel syndrome attack. It is not only the caffeine, but an enzyme that triggers the onset of IBS attack. Coffee is an acidic drink that will worsen the symptoms of irritable bowel syndrome.

2.   *Yoghurt:* Yoghurt is deemed to be good for health as it promotes the healthy bacteria in the digestive system. However, yoghurt is not a good option for those suffering from irritable bowel syndrome. Milk and milk products should be avoided by those suffering from IBS. The proteins and casein found in yoghurt are very difficult to digest and this will aggravate the conditions of irritable bowel syndrome.

3.   *Alcohol:* People consume alcohol during the evenings as it helps them to relax and unwind after a stressful day. However, it is not advisable for those suffering from irritable bowel syndrome to consume alcohol. Alcohol irritates the digestive tract and triggers symptoms of irritable bowel syndrome.

4.   *Vitamins:* People take vitamins to avoid IBS. However, not all vitamins are good for those suffering from irritable bowel syndrome. Some vitamins may be good while others may be bad for the system. It is best to consult your doctor for the best vitamins suited to your condition.

5.   *Avoiding vegetables and fruits:* This is one of the worst things that one can do. People assume that the insoluble fiber contained in fruits and vegetables will trigger an attack of IBS. Avoiding fruits and vegetables is an invitation to disease. Consuming both soluble and insoluble fiber can alleviate the symptoms of irritable bowel syndrome.

6.   ***Add soluble fiber to your diet:*** Soluble fiber is advertized to be a laxative and most persons with symptoms of irritable bowel syndrome neglect to take their soluble fiber supplements, thinking that these will worsen the conditions. Soluble fiber works as a stabilizing agent to minimize the symptoms of IBS.

7.   ***Soda:*** Carbonated drinks are bad for those suffering from irritable bowel syndrome. Doctors advise drinking plenty of water, but that does not include carbonated drinks. These will very often trigger symptoms of irritable bowel syndrome.

Irritable Bowel Syndrome Online

The Internet has become the largest source of information and is accessible to a large number of people in the recent times. From scientific information to cooking recipes from gardening to the latest gossips, all type of information is available on the internet. Therefore, finding information on Irritable Bowel Syndrome, online is not at all difficult.

However, since there is a vast amount of data available on the internet, it is better to streamline your search to the relevant data that you need. For this, you need to consider certain parameters, before starting the search:

1.   ***The kind of information required:*** Having a basic idea of the type of information that you need, will help to narrow down the search for irritable bowel syndrome. It could be some specific information like the symptoms of the disorder or the various treatments that are available for irritable bowel syndrome. You must also determine whether you want the medical or scientific information about the disorder or whether you need the general information that Is easy for the layperson to understand. Understanding the objective of the information will go a long way in avoiding wastage of time sifting through unwanted information. In this manner, you can visit the websites easily and quickly to get the information on irritable bowel syndrome that you require.

2.   ***The size of the information:*** You must also have an idea of the quantity of information you require. Some websites dealing with the subject matter have a larger amount of information than others. You can view the contents of the sites to decide whether or not it contains the data you need.

Once these parameters are decided upon, you can begin searching for information on irritable bowel syndrome, online. There are a few types of websites that may be useful in finding the information you need and these are mentioned below:

i)   ***Web Encyclopedias:*** These sites provide a wealth of knowledge on a variety of subjects and may be the best source to get information on irritable bowel syndrome, online. The sites are designed to provide easy access to those looking for information. Web encyclopedias provide information in a manner that everyone can understand easily. They have definitions and explanations for the subject matter and these are presented in a manner that can be easily understood by the common man.

How To Win Your War Against Irritable Bowel Syndrome

ii)   ***Support Groups:*** People who have experiences in irritable bowel syndrome launch these websites. These sites provide information regarding the treatments, symptoms and tips on coping with the ailment, or its prevention. These are sites that provide help to the persons who suffer from irritable bowel syndrome.

iii)   ***Medical Information Sites:*** Medical information sites provide a platform for the discussion of the disorder, in this case irritable bowel syndrome and also provide information on its treatment. They have the information on the latest developments and research done in the field of irritable bowel syndrome. A comprehensive medical knowledge is available to those seeking online information on irritable bowel syndrome.

iv)   ***Product sites:*** A range of products is available for the treatment of irritable bowel syndrome in the form of medicines and books. Most of these sites promise to alleviate the suffering caused due to irritable bowel syndrome. Besides this, these sites also contain general information relating to irritable bowel syndrome, its treatment and causes.

With the help of online searches for data on irritable bowel syndrome, one can be aware of the disorder and take steps towards a healthy lifestyle by changing the diet and practicing stress management.

<u>Constipation And Irritable Bowel Syndrome</u>

Constipation is a common complaint related to the digestive system. It varies with each individual and each person's bowel movements differ. In case of some, it may be hard stools, whereas for others it may be infrequent stools. There is straining as the stools are hard and painful to pass. There is also the general feeling of incomplete emptying of the bowels. In very severe cases of constipation, the bowels may be obstructed due to fecal impactions, preventing the passage of stools. Since there are various causes to constipation, different treatments are needed to solve the problems.

In case of persons suffering from irritable bowel syndrome, constipation alternates with diarrhea. There are no fixed numbers of bowel movements per week to be considered as normal. Infrequent bowel movement without any problems is not considered abnormal. Bowel movement three times in a day or a single regular bowel movement per day is considered as normal. Generally, as people advance in age, the number of bowel movement decreases.

About 50% of the population follows the common pattern of having one bowel movement per day. Most people do not have a similar number of bowel movement every day.

A person is considered to be suffering from constipation when he has three or less than three bowel movements in a week. Having only one bowel movement per week is considered a severe case of constipation. However, there is no medical justification for not feeling any serious discomfort even if there is no bowel movement in three consecutive days. There is no sign of accumulating toxins in the intestines due to infrequent bowel movements. Some persons may undergo mental stress in such cases.

Chronic constipation is associated with irritable bowel syndrome, though it does not require immediate treatment. There are no symptoms of rectal bleeding or inflammation of the lining in the abdomen so it is not a worrisome condition. Constipation is believed to be a symptom of irritable bowel syndrome.

How To Win Your War Against Irritable Bowel Syndrome

Bowel movements are controlled by the nervous system that controls the voluntary human activities. Constipation may result from the frequent suppression of the urge to exercise bowel movement.

Diet very often affects the activities of the intestinal tract and the digestive system. Therefore, change in a diet is recommended as a therapy for persons suffering from irritable bowel syndrome. Fiber rich food containing vegetables and fresh fruits helps to create bulky and soft stools thus relieving constipation. Five to six servings of natural fiber per day is ideal for a healthy bowel movement. Supplementary fibers also aid those who do not respond to natural fibers.

Constant use of stimulants and laxatives may cause constipation due to damage in the intestinal muscles. It is unclear whether the laxative caused the damage or the damage was present before their use. However, laxatives may be avoided as much as possible and if necessary, can be used with caution, or as a last resort for the treatment of irritable bowel syndrome.

Irritable Bowel Syndrome – General Information, Treatments And Causes

Irritable bowel syndrome (IBS) is a common functional disorder affecting the colon and is caused because the bowels do not function properly. Since it cannot be classified as a disease, there is no specific cure for it. The treatment is mostly symptomatic, and very often a slight change in diet and lifestyle can work wonders to keep the symptoms at bay. Although it does not require any surgery or operation, occasionally drugs may be used for the treatment.

A large number of people are affected by IBS and since it is a functional disorder, there are no physical changes or damage to the bowels. The problem arises due to the malfunctioning of the gastrointestinal tract, specifically the large intestine. In order to diagnose irritable bowel syndrome, one has to check for the symptoms. Symptoms of IBS may be present in the form of bloating, abdominal pain, constipation or diarrhea. Both constipation and diarrhea appear alternatively, in the sense that when diarrhea is suppressed, constipation may follow, thus making the treatment a little more complicated.

The doctor may use x-rays to study the interior of the colon. Barium enema is administered through the anus into the bowels which helps to show any abnormalities in the large intestine. This may help to treat any problems in the intestinal area, although the irritable bowel syndrome does not present anatomical complications.

Irritable bowel syndrome has no cure. The treatment is symptomatic and may involve changes in diet to include more fruits and vegetables to increase fiber content. The treatment may also involve relaxation and stress management techniques, along with medication for alleviating certain problematic conditions. What works best depends on the individual's condition.

Some types of foods trigger the symptoms of IBS. These include coffee, alcohol, milk products, cream-based products, chocolates, nuts and fried foodstuffs. Smoking also aggravates the irritable bowel syndrome. The person suffering from IBS can minimize the intake of these problematic food items and increase the natural fiber intake in their diet.

There may be some other food items that may trigger irritable bowel syndrome. In order to determine these, it is advisable to keep track of these foods. Keep a track of when the particular

How To Win Your War Against Irritable Bowel Syndrome

food item was consumed and what symptoms were triggered. This will help to determine the problem foods that trigger an attack of IBS for you. The best remedy would be to avoid these foods altogether.

Medications prescribed by the doctor should be strictly followed. The condition of irritable bowel syndrome may worsen if the dosage of medications is not followed. Stress management techniques may be followed for relieving stress and relaxing the body muscles including those of the intestinal tract. A combination of fiber rich diet, stress management and medication will help to alleviate the symptoms of irritable bowel syndrome and help you to lead a healthy life.

The Use Of Zelnorm To Treat Irritable Bowel Syndrome

Zelnorm is the only prescription drug that is approved by FDA for treating the symptoms of irritable bowel syndrome or IBS. It is prescribed for women suffering from IBS with constipation. Zelnorm works by speeding up the stool process and hence should not be used by those suffering from diarrhea.

Serotonin is a chemical that is produced by the body to regulate the digestive processes. A slow digestive tract is one cause of constipation or irritable bowel syndrome. The reason may be low levels of serotonin generation in the body. The Zelnorm drug performs the function of serotonin by coordinating the muscles in the digestive tract to speed up the digestive processes. This effectively relieves the irritable bowel syndrome with constipation.

Fiber supplements and common laxatives increase the eater content in the stools. This makes the stools soft and easy to excrete from the body thus relieving the symptoms of constipation. Zelnorm drug does not manipulate the stool content in any way, but It influences the movement of the digestive tract.

However, Zelnorm drug has certain disadvantages that need to be mentioned, which is given below:

• Zelnorm drug cannot be prescribed to men afflicted with irritable bowel syndrome. It can be used only by women suffering from IBS with constipation.

• It cannot be taken if the patient is suffering from diarrhea. Since Zelnorm speeds up the process of stool formation, the diarrhea will be worsened, making it very dangerous for the patient. It may leave the patient severely dehydrated or lower the blood pressure and may even cause death.

• Zelnorm drug should never be prescribed for children suffering from constipation.

There are a number of safer alternatives to the use of Zelnorm for treating irritable bowel syndrome along with constipation:

How To Win Your War Against Irritable Bowel Syndrome

1.   Intake of soluble fiber supplements in the diet of patients suffering from irritable bowel syndrome can relieve the problem. The soluble fiber supplements may be taken by patients suffering from either constipation or diarrhea.
2.   Use of herbal medicines like fennel or peppermint can alleviate symptoms of IBS. Fennel usually taken in the form of tea stabilizes the digestive process. It regulates the contractions of the small intestine and relaxes the gut.

Peppermint capsules are known to relieve symptoms of irritable bowel syndrome and may be taken even by children. The specially coated peppermint capsules pass through the stomach to release the peppermint oil only in the small intestine. Just like the soluble fiber, peppermint oil capsules can be taken by patients suffering from either diarrhea or constipation.

Zelnorm drug can be used as a last resort when all the alternative therapies fail to work. It may be an effective drug in treating the symptoms of irritable bowel syndrome, but it has to be used with extreme caution.

<u>What You Should Know About Irritable Bowel Syndrome</u>

Most persons suffering from irritable bowel syndrome are embarrassed to visit the doctor for treatment. That is because anything related to bowel movement makes people squeamish. Very few people consult a doctor in this regard, as most of them prefer to search the internet in a bid to solve their problem, by consulting with other people anonymously. Searching for a cure for IBS on the Internet may be helpful in many ways, but to ensure proper treatment it is advisable to visit a doctor who can help solve the issue.

The causes of irritable bowel syndrome are technically still unknown. It is considered a functional disorder as the large intestine or colon does not function as required, though there may be nothing wrong with it.

The symptoms of irritable bowel syndrome can be triggered due to many factors. Research has shown that stress has a big impact on the symptoms of irritable bowel syndrome and serves as a trigger for IBS. IBS was believed to be a psychosomatic disease in the early days. The mind influences how the syndrome affects the body. People having hyperacidity or heart burn are aware of the connection between digestion and stress. Stress causes the generation of peptic acid in the stomach, and persons under tremendous stress very often suffer from hyperacidity. Stress triggers chemical reactions in the digestive system, which cause irritable bowel syndrome.

Food is another factor that contributes to the irritable bowel syndrome. Eating the wrong type of food that does not agree with your digestive system can cause an attack of IBS. Some kinds of food may be good whereas others may worsen the situation. For example, eating a fiber rich diet can help to reduce the symptoms of IBS whereas eating pasta and white bread may prove to be detrimental to the symptoms of the illness. Persons suffering from IBS can categorize food into three groups, namely,

- Foods that do not affect the symptoms of IBS.
- Foods that trigger symptoms of irritable bowel syndrome
- Foods they are unsure about.

How To Win Your War Against Irritable Bowel Syndrome

It is therefore, advisable to consult with a specialist of a nutritional expert to find out the foods that you can eat without the fear of triggering an attack.

A variety of treatments is available to treat irritable bowel syndrome. One of them is to adhere to a diet prescribed by an expert. Medicines to alleviate the symptoms of IBS are also available.

Some people opt for alternative healing therapies. They feel that these are more effective as compared to the allopathic medicines available in the market today. One instance of alternative medicine is acupuncture, wherein some nerves are triggered to numb the pain in the body. This therapy clears the passage of energy through the body and encourages a balance of energy. Relaxation techniques and reiki are other examples of alternative therapies that may prove beneficial for IBS.

Diagnosis And Treatments For Irritable Bowel Syndrome

Information on the nature of a disease helps to look for better options for the treatment of that disease. Irritable Bowel Syndrome or IBS is one such disorder wherein the symptoms are very complex and providing the right kind of treatment becomes a challenge. It is a known fact that irritable bowel syndrome is a disorder generally related to the gastrointestinal tract, specifically related to the colon. It is not a serious disease, but can cause a lot of stress and disruption of normal activities for those suffering from it.

The first step in the diagnosis of IBS is to see your doctor a soon as you suspect that you may have the ailment. The doctor will diagnose the problem by looking at the medical history of the patient and classifying the symptoms as those pertaining to irritable bowel syndrome.

There are no specific tests to define irritable bowel syndrome. However, the doctor may conduct several tests to rule out the disease over other conditions. These tests may include blood tests, stool sample tests or x-rays. The doctor may perform a colonoscopy or a sigmoidoscopy on the patient. Colonoscopy is used for a close examination of the colon. A flexible tube with a small camera at the end is inserted into the anus of the patient. The image captured by the camera is projected on a screen which is used by the gastroenterologist for examination of the colon tissues.

However, colonoscopy by itself may not provide a solution to the problem. If the test results are negative, then the doctor will consider the other symptoms and diagnose your illness accordingly. He may enquire as to the frequency and intensity of the attacks, the stool consistency and changes in the bowel movements. Most doctors rely on a list of symptoms to classify the condition as irritable bowel syndrome.

On identifying the symptoms of IBS, treatment can be started to alleviate the condition. Persons suffering from a mild attack of irritable bowel syndrome may respond quickly to the treatment. However, chronic symptoms of IBS may be difficult to treat. The attack may subside with treatment but recur within a few days.

There is no cure for irritable bowel syndrome. However, treatments for the symptoms are available. Your physician may offer you advice on the best treatment suited to your condition.

How To Win Your War Against Irritable Bowel Syndrome

He may advise you to manage stress and generally change your lifestyle. Medications may be provided to relieve the symptoms as a part of a comprehensive therapy. The doctor may prescribe laxatives for constipation and anti- diarrheal medicines to control diarrhea. Antispasmodics are prescribed frequently to control muscle spasms and reduce abdominal pain. The disadvantages of antidepressants and antispasmodics are that they cause constipation. The doctor may prescribe relaxants to induce the bladder and intestines to relax. The medications are known to be addictive so they have to be used with caution.

Specific Medicines for treating irritable bowel syndrome are given below:

-       Lotronex (Alosetron hydrochloride): This medicine is recommended for women with symptoms of diarrhea where all other treatments have failed. There are severe side effects of the medicine in the form of constipation due to restricted blood flow to the colon.
-       Zelnorm(Tegaserod maleate): This is a short term treatment used for 4 to 6 weeks among women. The side effect of this drug is severe constipation.

It is absolutely necessary to follow the doctor's advice to the letter. Failing to follow the doctor's advice and guidelines may worsen the condition of irritable bowel syndrome.

What Is Irritable Bowel Syndrome?

Irritable Bowel Syndrome or IBS is a functional disorder that is related to the dysfunction of the large intestine also known as colon. IBS is not a life threatening disease like cancer or brain tumor, though it can disrupt the normal social life of the person suffering from it. It is termed as irritable bowel 'syndrome' because it involves a group of symptoms. Early identification of the disorder can help to take the necessary steps for alleviating the stressful symptoms.

Contrary to the common belief, irritable bowel syndrome is not classified as a disease, but is more of a functional disorder. The large intestine does not function properly and causes cramping in the abdominal area, bloating, gas constipation and diarrhea. This may be painful condition but does not cause any damage or inflammation to the bowels or the intestinal tract.

- ***Symptoms of IBS:***

Irritable bowel syndrome manifests in different ways in different people. Some of the symptoms are felt whereas others are evident in the stools of the patient. The patients feel pain or cramps in the abdominal area or a feeling of incomplete bowel movement. The patient may suffer from constipation or diarrhea. Bloated abdomen or mucous in the stool may be evident.

- ***How to diagnose IBS:***

Besides verifying the symptoms, the doctor may perform some tests to rule out any other disease that might have symptoms similar to that of IBS. The doctor may conduct medical tests like a blood test, physical exam or an x-ray of the bowel, commonly known as barium enema or lower GI series. Barium is a thick liquid that is passed into the bowel through the anus so that the interior of the bowels show up clearly on the x-rays. Another test is a colonoscopy that uses a thin tube with a camera attached to the end to see the insides of the intestines for detecting any problems.

- ***Tips to keep irritable bowel syndrome at bay:***

a) A change in diet is the easiest method to alleviate IBS. Avoid eating foods that trigger an attack of irritable bowel syndrome. Increase your natural fiber content by eating lots of fruit and vegetables.

b) Keeping note of the all the foods that cause an attack of IBS, so that they can be avoided.

How To Win Your War Against Irritable Bowel Syndrome

c)   Keep away from caffeine, sweeteners and alcohol as these cause the IBS to flare –up.
Avoid fatty foods like desserts, pastries and fried foodstuffs.

d)   The Premenstrual Syndrome (PMS) among women is known to cause irritable bowel
syndrome. This can be regulated with the help of the appropriate diet which in turn will control
IBS symptoms.

e)   Consultation with the doctor is essential before taking any steps for the treatment of
irritable bowel syndrome.

The irritable bowel syndrome is a common disorder prevalent among at least 20% of
Americans. It can be controlled by making dietary changes and practicing relaxation techniques.

<u>Common Irritable Bowel Syndrome Symptoms</u>

Irritable Bowel Syndrome or IBS is a functional disorder that is related to the dysfunction of the large intestine also known as colon. IBS is not a life threatening disease like cancer or brain tumor, though it can disrupt the normal social life of the person suffering from it. It can cause a great amount of stress to those suffering from it due to its peculiar symptoms. Early identification of the disorder can help to take the necessary steps for alleviating the stressful symptoms. Some information on the symptoms of irritable bowel syndrome is being discussed here.

During earlier times, it was not known whether there were any symptoms that could be attributed to irritable bowel syndrome. Therefore, the diagnosis would be a different disease altogether and the treatment would be ineffective. However, with a lot of research and studies on the subject, a group of specialists has established a set of standards to check out if the person has the symptoms of IBS.

ROME I, II and III criteria form the basis for the judging if what the person experiences constitutes symptoms of irritable bowel syndrome. The ROME II criteria diagnoses patients on the basis of data collected over a period of twelve weeks in the previous year. The ROME II classifies the abdominal pain suffered by patients into three categories as below:

I)   Pain that is relieved by having a bowel movement
II)   Pain with change in frequency of the bowel movement
III)   Pain with a change in the appearance of the stools

A change in the frequency of the bowel movement would mean a sudden abnormality in the bowel movement. This may be more than three times a day or less than three times a week. A sudden onset of abnormality of the bowel movement can be deemed to be irritable bowel syndrome.

Symptoms associated with irritable bowel syndrome can be quite contradictory in nature and confusing to a lot of people. Persons suffering from IBS may experience two kinds of symptoms and these are:

How To Win Your War Against Irritable Bowel Syndrome

- ***Diarrhea*** - This symptom constitutes very frequent bowel movements. The stools could be watery and loose and can also have mucus.
- ***Constipation*** - Constipation means having difficulty in passing stools. This is due to the stools being hard, lumpy, and difficult to excrete.

The symptoms of irritable bowel syndrome make life very uncomfortable for those suffering from the disorder. In some cases, the discomfort and pain may be so severe that the patients may absent themselves from work and avoid socializing. A common symptom of IBS is having gas or bloating in the abdominal area. Often, this gas is released by breaking wind.

A patient need not have all of these symptoms at once. The doctors usually conduct examinations to find out if the symptoms the patients experience are indeed irritable bowel syndrome.

It is important to be aware of the various symptoms that lead to irritable bowel syndrome. An early diagnosis and treatment can help to prevent this disorder from affecting the lifestyle of the individual. Awareness about the symptoms and knowing how to control these symptoms before they get out of hand is very crucial to leading a healthy and stress free life.

Understanding Irritable Bowel Syndrome

Most people live with the symptoms of irritable bowel syndrome (IBS) without being aware that it is a disorder. Hence they are surprised at being diagnosed for the ailment, or rather, surprised that the doctor has put a name to symptoms that they thought were normal occurrences. They have been suffering for several years with the symptoms and experiences like abdominal cramping or bloating happen so often that it becomes a normal occurrence in their perception. People get used to these discomforts and may tend to ignore it.

Irritable bowel syndrome is the most common disorder diagnosed by gastroenterologists. About 15 to 20% of the American population suffers from irritable bowel disorder. Many people experience mild abdominal discomfort that lead to aches in the abdominal muscles. This may be followed by a phase where there is no abdominal discomfort. Irritable bowel syndrome is also known as mucous colitis, spastic colitis, spastic colon, nervous stomach or irritable colon. The symptoms include abdominal pain, cramps, bloating, constipation or diarrhea. This is a disorder related to the gastrointestinal tract, more so to the large intestine or colon.

Irritable bowel syndrome is classified as a functional disorder and cannot be diagnosed with the conventional methods of blood tests and x-rays. It is possible to diagnose it only by a careful examination of the physiological functions. At times colonoscopy is used for a close examination of the colon. A flexible tube with a small camera at the end is inserted into the anus of the patient. The image captured by the camera is projected on a screen which is used by the gastroenterologist for examination of the colon tissues. However, colonoscopy by itself may not provide a solution to the problem.

IBS is a complicated condition and very often difficult to diagnose. It is believed to be caused due to the disturbance in the interaction between the intestines, the autonomic nervous system, responsible for control of the lining of the intestinal tract and the brain. It is distinguished by various symptoms of abdominal discomfort, change in bowel patterns, watery stools or constipation. Each person experiences varied symptoms where some may have mild attacks while others may have severely disabling ones.

There is no cure for irritable bowel syndrome; patients can be treated symptomatically. Changes in lifestyles, diet, reduction of stress and some medication may help to alleviate symptoms.

How To Win Your War Against Irritable Bowel Syndrome

Again, it all depends on the individual's bodily constitution. Some persons may respond to treatment while others may not. Eating the right type of food and including fiber in the diet may help to keep the symptoms at bay. It is best to seek medical help to treat the disorder and to formulate a diet plan suitable to the individual needs, with the help of a dietician.

Treatments For Irritable Bowel Syndrome

Irritable Bowel syndrome or IBS is a disorder affecting the gastrointestinal tract. Although the origins of this disorder are unknown, the symptoms include bloating abdominal pain, gas, diarrhea, cramps and constipation. The treatment can be symptomatic to alleviate the symptoms. There are various methods of treating irritable bowel syndrome. These are listed below:

- ***Changing the diet:***

IBS is a disorder mainly related to the bowel movements of the individual. Most people change their diet because they may experience constipation or diarrhea. However, it is advisable to consult the doctor before making dietary changes. Certain foods trigger an IBS attack and doctors are the right people to provide this advice. For instance if you try to diagnose the condition on your own, you may mistake lactose intolerance for Irritable bowel syndrome.

- ***Treatment:***

There are some patients who continuously suffer from IBS. They require treatment or therapy for taking care of the problem. Eating fiber rich foods is often recommended to those afflicted by irritable bowel syndrome. Fiber helps to expand the digestive tract and reduce the possibility of a spasm when food is being digested. Eating fibrous foods promotes regular and easy bowel movement and prevents constipation. Fiber can be added slowly to the diet to prevent other complications.

Stress is known to trigger symptoms of irritable bowel syndrome. Therefore many doctors advise stress management and relaxation techniques to patients afflicted by IBS. Maintaining a food journal to jot down the foods that caused an IBS attack can help to avoid those food items. This may help to prevent future attacks of irritable bowel syndrome. Smoking is injurious to health and more so, to those having irritable bowel syndrome. Patients that smoke are advised to quit smoking for their own health.

- ***Medications:***

Antispasmodic medicines are prescribed for patients suffering from IBS. This helps to control or slow down the digestive tract to decrease spasms. Each individual will react to medicines in different ways. What may be working with one may not work for others.

How To Win Your War Against Irritable Bowel Syndrome

Anti-Diarrhea medication is prescribed to those suffering from loose bowel movement. Over-the- counter anti- diarrhea medicines are available without doctor's prescriptions. Us of these medicines for simple diarrhea may work, but not for IBS. It is better to consult the doctor in such cases.

Anti depressants in small doses may be effective in controlling IBS. In the recent years, new types of medicines are specially made for people who are allergic to anti depressants.

It is always advisable to consult the doctor before taking any medication. Self medication is risky to say the least, and should never be practiced.

What Is Irritable Bowel Syndrome

The term 'Irritable Bowel Syndrome' (IBS) brings to mind the idea that it is serious disease. Many are puzzled as to what the illness is and wonder about its symptoms. However, in actual fact it is a disorder and a condition where the bowels do not function properly. This disorder may not be caused by any factors but it is a dysfunction of the bowels. The non-functioning of the bowels then lead to various symptoms that a person may experience. In order to fully understand irritable bowel syndrome, one should be aware of some of the factors that contribute to this disorder and they are:

1. **Symptoms**

Symptoms are the common signs of irritable bowel syndrome in humans. The symptoms give an idea of how irritable bowel syndrome affects the body. It is a collection of symptoms that manifest in the body to show that the bowels are not functioning properly. A person suffering from IBS may experience abdominal pain, bloating, constipation or diarrhea.

2. **Causes**

As explained earlier, irritable bowel syndrome is a disorder of the bowels. Researchers have not yet found out the exact causative factors for irritable bowel syndrome. However, some people have the misconception that irritable bowel syndrome is the result of consuming food items that do not agree with their digestion. Yet others misconstrue it to be caused by some sort of bacteria or virus.

3. **Triggers**

There are varieties of factors that serve as triggers to irritable bowel syndrome; the two main triggers are given below:

- **Stress**

Research has shown that stress has a big impact on the symptoms of irritable bowel syndrome. Any form of stress including being diagnosed for IBS can trigger the symptoms. Therefore, counseling for stress management is an integral part of the treatment for IBS. Alternative therapies are used for the treatment of IBS. Yoga and acupuncture are some of the alternate therapies used to relieve stress and consequently the symptoms of irritable bowel syndrome.

- **Food**

Consuming the wrong kind of food can trigger IBS symptoms. Foods high in fat content and alcohol, are known triggers for IBS, and hence should be avoided by those suffering from the ailment.

4.   Treatments

People suffering from irritable bowel syndrome have a sensitive colon that reacts to some kinds of food, medicines or stress. Treatment of Irritable bowel syndrome involves medications and alternative therapies, along with a change in diet. The use of drugs to reduce the symptoms of IBS is prevalent today and since stress is a causative factor, relieving stress is also important to control the symptoms. A person suffering from Irritable bowel syndrome has to make efforts to keep the symptoms at bay. Diet control and relaxation techniques will help to alleviate the symptoms of irritable bowel syndrome.

How To Win Your War Against Irritable Bowel Syndrome

This Product Is Brought To You By

DAVID A OSEI